WOULD YOU LIKE TO HAVE A MEMORY LIKE GOOGLE?

Have you tried the tricks other memory books teach and given up? Can you actually improve your memory? What does science say?

Memory researcher Jeremy Genovese knows there's good news — science offers real help. A growing body of research has given us tools and techniques for REAL memory improvement. Unfortunately, most people are unaware of the science of peak memory. Dr. Genovese's book bridges that gap.

Remembering Willie Nelson: The Science of Peak Memory introduces a number of ideas accepted by memory scientists, but largely unknown outside the laboratory. In easy-to-understand language, Dr. Genovese explains how you can harness these ideas to dramatically improve your memory.

What would a better memory mean for you? Better grades? A better income? Not forgetting someone's name? Remembering where you parked?

What would a mind like Google mean to you?

REMEMBERING WILLIE NELSON

The Science of Peak Memory

Jeremy E.C. Genovese, Ph.D

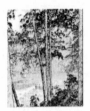

Moonshine Cove Publishing, LLC

Abbeville, South Carolina U.S.A.

ISBN: 978-1-937327-569
Library of Congress Control Number: 2014957367

Book cover and interior design by Moonshine Cove staff; cover image public domain

DEDICATION

For Teresa, With Love

ACKNOWLEDGEMENTS

I owe a deep debt of gratitude to my many friends and colleagues at Cleveland State University, particularly those in the Department of Curriculum and Foundations. My department chair Maruis Boboc deserves special mentions for his support and forbearance over the several years I spent on this project. Also, I would like to thank our superb departmental staff, Rosalyn Adams and Sharon Jefferson.

This book would not have been possible without my wife Teresa Kammerman, to whom I owe everything.

About the Author

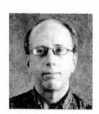

Dr. Jeremy Genovese, Ph.D, teaches educational psychology, human development, and learning theory at the College of Education and Human Services at Cleveland State University. An active researcher, he has published papers on human learning, individual differences, and evolutionary psychology. His papers have appeared in such journals as *Personality and Individual Differences*, *Evolutionary Psychology*, *The Journal of Educational Research*, and *The Journal of Genetic Psychology*. Most recently he has been working in Cleveland State University Human Performance Laboratory studying the effects of exercise on cognitive function.

Dr. Genovese lives in Beachwood, Ohio with his wife Teresa Kammerman, MD. They have two adult children.

He blogs about memory and related topics at http://peakmemory.me/

REMEMBERING
WILLIE NELSON

Chapter 1

Forgetting Willie Nelson

Some people say I have a good memory. They are mistaken, and I can prove it. I once forgot Willie Nelson, or rather I forgot his name. For the life of me, I could not recover the name of the famous rebel country singer. In my mind, I could remember what he looked like; I could recall his voice in several songs. I even remembered he starred in the movie *The Electric Horseman*, with Robert Redford and sang the song "Mammas Don't Let Your Babies Grow Up To Be Cowboys" but I just could not call up his name.

We often don't know why we forget. But in this case I blame Woody Starr. You see, when I forgot Willie Nelson's name I was sure it was Woody's fault. Woody is an unforgettable character who lives at the Chautauqua Institution in western New York, where I spend my summers. So unforgettable, an extreme extrovert with long hair and a cowboy hat, all the local postal workers know him and he has no problem receiving mail simply addressed to Woody, Chautauqua, New York.

One day Woody stopped me, he stops everyone, and showed me a photograph of himself with Willie Nelson. He told me Willie was a great human being and recommended I read his book the *Tao of Willie*. I trace my memory failure to this encounter. Now when I try to call up Willie's name I often get stuck on Woody's.

I was experiencing what psychologists call a tip of the tongue state, the inability to recall a piece of information with the accompanying sense we actually do know. These states are both frustrating and embarrassing. They are sometimes called "senior moments" and their increasing occurrence reminds us of our aging and our mortality. It seems inexplicable that we cannot recover information when we need it. To our surprise the information will sometimes come to us later without any effort, it just pops into mind; strong evidence the information was there all along, but we were simply unable to locate it. Frequently, we sense what we are looking for and feel blocked by some similar information. In this case my association between Willie and Woody, two names that sound similar, made it hard for me to retrieve Willie's name.

Tip of the tongue states are not the only frustrations we have with memory. Why can't we remember where we put the keys or parked the car? Will we recall the material we studied when we take the exam? Why do we have so much trouble matching the face with the name? What was the title of that great book we read?

I wrote this book because our situation is far from hopeless. I have learned through personal experience and academic research that there are ways we can improve memory and keep our brains active and engaged as we grow older. We do not need to surrender to inevitable senility, we can take positive action.

I've also seen firsthand the tragedy of dementia. As

a student, I conducted field research with dementia patients in a nursing home and witnessed the devastating consequence of memory loss. As the population ages, we face a tidal wave of Alzheimer's disease. The techniques described in this book may reduce your risk of dementia. I hope to convince you of the benefits of memory training and cognitive engagement. I hope more people will be able to live longer with their memories intact.

When people tell me I have a good memory I correct them and say "no I have a trained memory." There clearly are people who learn faster than others and people with extraordinary powers of recall. Examples of powerful memories include Solomon Shereshevsky, who could recall long strings of random digits 15 years after hearing them only once, and Kim Peek, a savant who could remember everything he read and was the model for the title character in the film *Rain Man*.

I am not one of these people and, I suspect, neither are you. However, it is likely you have a perfectly good memory you could learn to use much more efficiently. This is a possible because a science of memory has emerged that gives us new insight into how information is acquired, retained, and recalled. It is now within our power to put this science into service of an improved memory.

I have been interested in memory improvement since my early teens. The first memory improvement book I ever read was *10 Days to a Successful Memory* by Dr. Joyce Brothers and Edward Egan.[1] I was, at that time, a struggling junior high school student and I recognized that a better memory might make school easier. Unfortunately, the book was a disappointment. It did tell a great story; how Dr. Brothers memorized enough information about the sport of boxing to win the top prize on the 1950s quiz show *The $64,000 Question*. Unfortunately, most of the advice didn't seem to help much, and I don't think I actually finished reading it.

Over time I read other memory improvement books, such as *The Memory Book* by Harry Lorayne and Jerry Lucas,[2] and found the mnemonic strategies they advocated were helpful, but of limited application.

Later, while pursuing my doctorate, I came to the scientific study of memory. Reading across several sub-disciplines of psychology, educational, developmental, cognitive, and behavioral, I realized that real progress has been made in our understanding of how memory works and how it could be improved. The goal of this book is to teach you how to train your memory. I believe this kind of brain exercise is no less important than physical exercise for our bodies. The training advocated in this book will help you with everyday memory issues and, yes, there is evidence it may reduce your risks of dementia.

We Are Our Memories

Our survival depends on our ability to locate ourselves in time and space. We synthesize information from our senses to map our position in the three-dimensional world of space, but to locate ourselves in the fourth dimension of time we need powers of memory and anticipation. Memory holds our sense of continuity in life. It retains hard lessons learned and the material for agreeable nostalgia. It allows us to reflect on the turning points in our lives and recollect both the sweet and the bitter. It tells us friend from enemy and holds the names of our kin. It is the repository of the skills that allow us to make a living and ride a bicycle. It is where our beliefs, illusions, regrets, accomplishments, ambitions, and inclinations are stored. When poet John Donne wondered "where all past years are," he invoked the powerful mystery of time and memory. Our past exists only in our memory and, to some large extent, we are our memories.

Frau Auguste D. was a patient of the psychiatrist Alois Alzheimer. She was the first individual identified with the form of dementia that now bears the name Alzheimer's. As her memory failed she voiced our deepest fear; "I have lost myself."[3]

It is this identity of self and memory that makes forgetting so frightening. As we age we worry about decline into dementia, where the damaged brain fails even elementary memory tasks. People with Alzheimer's disease frequently do not know where they are, cannot recognize loved ones, and often inhabit a world of confusion and despair.

As life expectancy increases, so does the number of people diagnosed with dementia. It is likely every reader has encountered someone suffering from clinical memory loss. We cannot help but worry that this could be our fate. We examine ourselves for evidence of decline. Did we forget our keys again? Did we forget the name of the last book we read? Have I told this story before, and will I be seen as an aging bore by people too kind to tell me they have heard it all before?

Memory does become more difficult with age. This book does not promise impossible miracles, but we need not be complacent or defeatist. We would not expect our older bodies to have the same athletic prowess as in our twenties. Yet, despite our physical decline we still see the value in exercise. Exercise slows the pace of aging and is protective against many of the forces of mortality. Exercise will not give us unending youth, but it will improve the quality of our lives. The message of this book is that the use of memory strategies and memory training can produce real benefits. We can continue to learn and even improve our memories into old age, we can stave off or, at least moderate, many of the cognitive effects of the aging process. Just like physical exercise, it will take a commitment to regular daily work, but the payoffs are high, and it is worth the effort.

Lest you think this claim is hyperbole, let me give you the example of Akira Haraguchi who at age 61 set the world record for memorizing digits of pi; he successfully recited 100,000 digits in 16.5 hours. The digit sequence of pi is random with no order or known pattern, and it is a popular test of superior memory performance.

Haraguchi denies having any special power of memory. He told one interviewer "I'm certainly no genius, I'm just an ordinary old guy." In addition, Haraguchi believes that memory can actually improve with age:

When you are young, you look at the sky and think it's a nice day. Then you might think, "I might as well go driving." When you grow older, however, you start observing the sunlight and its reflection on leaves. You develop the ability to imagine more, which helps you associate things . . . A whole new different way of memorizing things becomes available when you get older.[4]

Memorization of the digits of pi is, undoubtedly, an arcane pursuit. Yet by studying the techniques used by memory athletes like Haraguchi we have learned a lot about strategies to improve memory. Some of these techniques, called mnemonics, will be described in this book. But this is not just a book about mnemonics, this is a book about memory training as the key to brain training.

What Lies Ahead

The message of brain training has reached the public. We are told to keep our minds engaged to reduce our risk of dementia. This is good advice. Unfortunately, the type of brain training that has been widely advocated is probably not demanding enough to have much of an effect. Completing a daily sudoku puzzle is simply not enough.

In subsequent chapters, I will review the evidence for the benefits of brain training and suggest foreign language learning as an ideal approach to brain training. I will introduce you to the notion of spaced repetition, mnemonics, and the testing effect and explain how to use computer software to harness these effects.

Finally, I will outline a plan of daily memory training using spaced repetition software to help you avoid tip of the tongue forgetting and keep your memory strong.

---

1 Brohters, J. & Eagan, E. P. F. (1957). *10 days to a successful memory*. Englewood Cliff, NJ: Prentice-Hall.
2 Lorayne, H. & Lucas, J. (1974). *The memory book*. New York: Ballantine Books.
3 Shenk, D. (2003). *The forgetting: Alzheimer's: Portrait of an epidemic*. New York: Anchor Books.
4 Otake, T. (2006, December, 2006). How can anyone remember 100,000 numbers? *Japan Times*. [http://search.japantimes.co.jp/print/fl20061217x1.html]

Chapter 2

A Case for Memory

Everyone seems to want a better memory. Given the demand for memory improvement, it might seem strange or unnecessary to have to make a case for memory.

Yet memory has been under attack from a number of quarters. In popular culture, in political circles, and, most surprising of all, among some educators, memory is often dismissed as unnecessary and even harmful. American culture has strong anti-intellectual undertones that values street smarts over book knowledge and dismisses factual knowledge as trivia.[1] Memory is even held, by some, to be a distraction from learning and seen as detrimental to higher order skills, such as creativity or critical thinking.

This anti-memory bias is reflected in oft repeated admonition "you don't need to know that, you can always look it up." Teachers are told to focus on the higher order skills and avoid those onerous memory tasks. For example, Alfie Kohn, a popular writer on education, claims "committing things to memory may train you to be a better memorizer, but there is absolutely no reason to think that it provides any real cognitive benefits."[2]

So memory does need a defense and I am prepared to offer one here.

It has been suggested, that schools should downplay memorization and concentrate on higher order thinking. Kohn also wrote, "if school is based on the 'bunch o' facts' model for long enough, our children may be less likely to develop the skills and dispositions of critical thinking."[3]

Along a similar line, educational researchers David Berliner and Bruce Biddle argued:

> America needs citizens who are flexible, who embrace new ideas, who can reason well when faced with complex ideas, and who are capable of self-directed learning. It is difficult to understand how citizens with these skills and interests are likely to develop if our high schools merely pump concrete bits of knowledge from the past into passive students.[4]

If we ignore the fact that Berliner and Biddle contradict themselves a page later and argue that "it is *necessary* that students have an appropriate knowledge base"[5] (emphasis in the original) we can see there are a number of unexamined assumptions here; that flexibility and new ideas operate in a zero-sum competition with knowledge, and that concrete knowledge is only acquired passively. There is reason to doubt both these claims.

This assertion that memory comes at the expense of critical reasoning skills is seriously mistaken. One source of this belief appears to arise from a misunderstanding of Benjamin Bloom's distinction between higher and lower cognitive skills. In 1956 Bloom, a respected educational psychologist, proposed a systematic classification of educational goals. The system he and his colleagues created has had great influence both in educational measurement and instructional planning. Bloom proposed that educational objectives could be organized in a hierarchy of six categories:

1 Knowledge
2 Comprehension
3. Application
4. Analysis
5. Synthesis
6. Evaluation[6]

Over time this ordering has come to be regarded as a value judgment. The first category, knowledge, is often described as counterposed to categories two through six the higher levels of learning. For example, an article in the journal *Educational Leadership* tells us that

educators are adept at focusing on memorization of facts. Common examples include multiplication tables, spelling, and sets of principles in different subjects. However, an overemphasis on such procedures leave the learner impoverished, does not facilitate the transfer of learning and probably interferes with the development of understanding.[7]

In this view, knowledge is seen as debased and debasing. Bloom, however, was clear that the distinction between lower and higher skills was not a value judgment and that we need both sets of skills. He saw these levels of education as cumulative with higher skills resting on lower level accomplishments; "as we have defined them, the objectives in one class are likely to make use of and build on the behaviors found in the preceding classes in this list."[8]

Research supports Blooms contention, suggesting that higher order skills require strong background knowledge. In several path breaking studies, Barbara Hayes-Roth and Carol Walker found that people who committed facts to memory demonstrated greater ability to reason about those facts than individuals who had free access to the same information in text form.[9] These researchers found evidence of differences between how we search for information stored in written text and how we search for information stored in memory. When the information needed to solve a higher order problem is stored in text, we first need to extract the relevant facts. Then we need to compare all possible configurations of those facts. Using this procedure we soon exhaust our brain's processing capacity.

To understand this we need to think about the mathematics of combination. Imagine a child building a tower with four blocks each of a different color. Let's say red, white, blue, and green. We would like to know how many different four block towers the child could build. For the first block of any tower, there are four possible colors to choose. By virtue of choosing one block, there will be only 3 colors to choose from for the second block. The way to figure out the total number of arrangements is to multiply together the number of choices at each step. So this would be $4 \times 3 \times 2 \times 1$, which equals 24. Mathematicians call this procedure the factorial and it is represented by a number followed by an exclamation point. Thus, if the child had 5 blocks the number of possible combinations would be $5! = 5 \times 4 \times 3 \times 2 \times 1 = 120$. One feature of the factorial is that the number of possible arrangements grows rapidly. If you had to arrange only ten blocks, there would be 3,628,800 possible different orderings.

The point here is that a simple procedure can generate enormous numbers of combinations. Think of the game of chess. While the rules of the game are finite and played with 32 pieces on 64 squares, the number of possible games is estimated to be about ten to the power of 120; that is one followed by 120 zeros.[10]

Similarly a small set of facts related by some finite set of rules may be able to form an unthinkably large number of potential connections. Trying to examine each one of the exploding number of combinations would soon swamps our brain's limited processing capacity.

Hayes-Roth and Walker pointed out that asked to solve a logic problem from text, a computer might compare exhaustively every possible logical configuration of facts. While within the capacity of a powerful computer, it is a feat beyond human processing ability. They conclude that "simply reading relevant texts for familiarization and then referring to them as needed provides an inadequate basis for deductive logic."[11] How is it, then, that we are able to reason about text? We solve the problem by storing acquired information in our long term memory based on logical associations.

If we compare the chess expertise of computers and humans we can see this difference in action. Chess computers do well because they can exhaustively compare the strengths of many alternative moves. Human chess experts cannot do this; they rely, instead, on their mastery of the underlying logic of the game, and the many games they have committed to memory. They are able to hold this information in long term memory because, after thousands of hours of play, they have internalized the logical structure of the game. This is one of the major differences between expert and novice players. Chess grand masters understand the board positions because the information they store in memory is structured in a way that reflects the relationships of pieces. Not only do they know more chess games than beginning player, they also have superior memory for board positions.[12] For chess players, as for expert performers in many fields, memory and skill are bound together in a tight reciprocal relationship.

In general, when information is stored in memory it is retained in a network of associations that, to some, extent already reflects the logical relationships between the facts. Hayes-Roth and Walker suggest that "once learned, pairs of critical facts are likely to be have been stored in *integrated* memory representations"[13] These authors conclude "apparently, learning the individual facts that are involved in a complex knowledge structure is an important, and perhaps necessary, precursor to a thorough understanding of the relationships among those facts."[14]

In order to retrieve information from long term memory, there must be some kind of search process. We do not examine every fact randomly until we hit upon the correct one; memory must have a structure and a search procedure.[15] Facts in our memory are already associated by their logical structure, and recalling one fact increases the probability of remembering a logically associated fact. When we try to solve problems with an insufficient knowledge base, the facts we look-up are isolated from each other and we are forced into an inefficient and, often, ineffective strategy of combining and comparing.

There is an irony here. Memory in education is often dismissed as the memorization of unconnected facts. Yet it is through memory that we find meaning in information by associating new information into our mental networks. It is precisely when we have to look everything up that we are faced with the problem of unconnected facts in uncertain relations. As Ralph Waldo Emerson pointed out "what was an isolated, unrelated belief or conjecture, our later experience instructs us how to place in just connection with other views which confirm and expand it." [16]

Imagine that you had to find the meaning of the word from a dictionary whose words were arranged randomly. You would be forced to look at each word sequentially until you found the one you were seeking. Fortunately, the dictionary is arranged in an order that allows you to quickly find the unknown word.[17] It is worth noting that to find information in the dictionary you must already hold in your memory the rules of alphabetization, otherwise the volume might as well be random.

Efforts to create artificial intelligence have also demonstrated the importance of factual knowledge. Both humans and intelligent machines perform better when they have the relevant background knowledge. [18] John Sweller, Emeritus Professor of Education at the University of New South Wales, has written that "competent problems solvers in a given area were competent because they had stored an enormous amount of information in long term memory."[19] One of the central problems for artificial intelligence computing is finding ways to build, organize, and access large amounts of background knowledge.

As author Susan Jacoby points out "without memory, judgments are made on the unsound basis of the most recent bit of half-digested information."[20]

One clear finding that has emerged from the research on memory is that meaningful material is easier to remember than information without meaning. Your ability to remember new material is facilitated if you can establish associations with material that you already know. For example, If I asked you to repeat *"ua mau ke ea o ke aina i ka pono"* after one hearing you would probably find it difficult. On the other hand, I suspect you would have no trouble repeating "many diamonds scintillate." Both phrases use 23 letters from the English alphabet. But in order to repeat a sentence you must first hold it, at least temporarily, in memory. For English speakers the second phrase is meaningful, we know each word individually and understand the message of the sentence as a whole. The first sentence is in the Hawaiian language, it is the motto of the state of Hawaii and means "the life of the land is perpetuated in righteousness." If you speak the Hawaii language, that is, if you are able to find meaning in those words, you would have no difficulty repeating the phrase.[21]

Psychologists often define meaningfulness as how well new information associates with existing knowledge.[22] Research has show that if you have deep knowledge of an area it is easier to remember new information about that subject.

One of the most difficult laboratory tests of memory is remembering numbers paired with words. In these tests, pairs of words and numbers are presented at rate of one pair every two seconds. The volunteers are then given one member of the pair and asked to recall the other. Performance is typically quite poor. Yet the difficult task is routinely performed by sports fans who easily remember the scores of many specific games. They can successfully recall the score when cued with the name of a specific game. In fact, there is a relationship between knowledge about a sport and the ability to remember scores. More knowledgeable fans have better memories for scores.[23]

This is not a new observation. Psychologist and philosopher William James, in a series of lectures delivered in 1892, noted that "a college athlete, who remains a dunce at his books, may amaze you by his knowledge of the 'records' at various feats and games, and provide himself a walking dictionary of sporting statistics." For the athlete, sports statistics form "not so many odd facts, but a concept system, so they stick"[24] Before James, Emerson noted "Tomorrow, when I know more, I recall that piece of knowledge and use it better."[25]

The point is that rich background knowledge makes it easier to remember new material.

Psychologist Gabriel Radvansky tells us that memory improves as the amount of information it contains grows. She compares it to a key collection: "the more keys you have, the more locks you can open."[26]

This is true, not only for sports, but for many critical areas of life. Remembering a doctor's advice and instructions can have real medical consequences. More knowledgeable patients have better memory of doctor's instructions than less knowledgeable patients.[27]

All this suggests that the common belief about memory, that you do not need to memorize anything that you can easily look-up, is deeply misguided. Knowledge builds on knowledge. Knowing facts about the world, knowing background, history, and context improves memory. Psychologist James Weinland pointed out:

> Memory is in one respect like money. The more money one has, the more interest it earns, which increases the capital and earns still more money. The more memories one accumulates, the more easily new memories are accumulated, which increases one's memory capital and earn more memory interest. Memories breed memories.[28]

Experimental research supports Weinland's contention. Another technique used by psychologists to study memory is called the word pair association task. Here an individual is given a set of word pairs to learn such as "zebra — horizon." Later the person will be given one member of the word pair and asked to recall the other. The ability to recall the missing word depends on the quantity and quality of the associations the individual is able to establish between the two words. As researcher Patrick Kyllonen, and his colleagues pointed out:

because relations between two paired-associate terms are constructed by drawing on previously stored facts, the breadth of factual knowledge an individual brings to the learning situation might be expected at least partly to determine paired-associate learning success. A learner with a rich network of facts stored in long-term memory will be able to retrieve numerous diverse facts related to each term. The more facts retrieved, the more likely that the learner will be able to construct a relation between terms. Further, with a richer knowledge base, a relation constructed will be more likely to be a distinctive relation, which will also contribute to memorability. A learner with an impoverished knowledge base, on the other hand, will be less likely to retrieve facts during study that will be useful for creating linking relations. Any relations constructed are likely to be poorer quality, that is less distinctive, than those constructed from a richer knowledge base. [29]

Education based only on memorization of facts would be barren; a curriculum based only on higher order skills is not possible. Psychologist Robert Sternberg wrote "to think critically, you need first to have content about which to think. Content in the absence of thinking is inert and meaningless; but thinking in the absence of content is vacuous."[30]

Fluency

The ability to respond automatically to lower level questions frees up capacity for other types of cognitive processes. An algebra student who has not mastered basic math facts is at an extreme disadvantage. Fluency in basic skills is a prerequisite for achievement at higher levels of education.[31]

The requirements of foreign language learning make a mockery of the claim that memory should play a limited role in education. Of course, you could look-up a word in a foreign language dictionary every time you needed it or try to rely on Google translations. But few would seriously think these strategies could replace the need to learn foreign languages.

The goal of most language learners is fluency. Fluency is ability to retrieve information from memory quickly. One the first things taught of any foreign language is the number system and new learners, with some effort, are able to master counting in the new language. However, these learners will often fail in even simple real word situations involving numbers such as making change. This is because they lack fluency with the newly learned number system. Fluency is a basic memory skill.[32]

Fluency in language requires a large vocabulary and the ability to call up information quickly. The critics of memory would doom us to a monolingual isolation. Howard Gardner reminds us that while language instruction would be "pointless" without "the opportunity to use the language productively — for reading, writing, or speaking." He acknowledges that "without question, many aspects of foreign language study can — and some must — be acquired by routine drill."[33]

While rote learning is often condemned, learning by repetition remains an unavoidable part of foreign language learning. Having said this, however, the science of memory has shown us that repetition can be made much more effective and far less burdensome. As we will see factors such as the spacing, number, and type of repetition can be manipulated to improve learning.[34]

As your second language vocabulary grows it becomes easier to learn new words in that language. The growing vocabulary creates more opportunities for associating new words. In addition, as you learn more words you come to recognize structural similarities between words, which, in turn, facilitates additional learning.[35] In other words, memorization facilitates new learning.

The Two Englishes

While the case for deliberate memorization may be clear for learning a second language, what is its role in learning English vocabulary? While it is true that we learn much of our vocabulary from context, rather than explicit instruction, it may still be that many English speakers would benefit from direct instruction of English vocabulary.[36]

This is because English is a diglossic language, in the sense that it contains two vocabularies. In a diglossic language, at least two versions of the language exist, each associated with different positions in the social hierarchy. In some cases, such as English, the language contains two vocabularies that reflect social stratification, with one acting as the language of ordinary people and common interaction and the other vocabulary being the words of prestige and power.

A number of languages are diglossic. For example, Hindi-Urdu, sometimes called Hindustani, is a diglossic language spoken on the Indian subcontinent. The name Hindi-Urdu identifies the two dialects of the same language. Hindi and Urdu share many words and essentially the same grammar. While they have different writing systems, for everyday conversations they are effectively the same and Urdu and Hindi speakers can communicate without difficulty. However, when one wants to discuss topics outside of ordinary interactions, say education, economics, or science, the languages diverge substantially. That is because their higher vocabularies draw on different sources. The higher vocabulary for Hindi comes from the ancient liturgical language of Hinduism; Sanskrit. While Urdu's higher vocabulary comes from Persian and Arabic. [37]

Arabic itself is also a diglossic language with an everyday dialect and literary dialect. Research has found that for many Arabic speakers learning the literary dialect is, in some ways, like learning a foreign language. The Arabic of the schools and books is different from the Arabic of home and this may contribute to lower levels of academic achievement.[38]

English also can be said to have two vocabularies both rooted in its historical development. Anglo-Saxon English was established in England by the early Germanic invaders. Latin words were introduced more slowly beginning with the Roman invasion and continuing as a consequence of the spread of Christianity. A major shift occurred with the Norman conquest of England in 1066. The Normans spoke a dialect of French that became the language of the ruling class. This meant that the British aristocracy spoke a Latinate language while the common people spoke Anglo-Saxon English, a Germanic language.

This division still persists in our vocabulary. There is an English that everyone learns to speak, this is the English of everyday interactions and its origins lie in Anglo-Saxon English. There is also an academic English, the English of science, literature, and education. This English is largely Latin and Greek in origin and includes words that were imported into English from the Norman Conquest and, later, during the Renaissance.[39] This difference is illustrated by two great works of English, both written around the same time, the King James Bible and the works of Shakespeare.

The King James Bible was written in Anglo-Saxon English, and while it was originally published in 1611 it is still largely comprehensible to most native English speakers. Indeed, it remains the preferred Bible for many Protestant churches.

Shakespeare, on the other hand, is a Renaissance author and students often find his writing difficult. Many English words borrowed from Latin and Greek are first recorded in his plays.[40]

Some linguists believe the Renaissance was the greatest period of vocabulary growth in the English language, primarily because of the importation of Graeco-Latinate words.

Educational arrangements in Elizabethan England served to perpetuate class distinctions in language. Schools for the poor and lower classes, when they existed at all, taught only the rudiments of reading and writing in the Anglo-Saxon English, while schools for the children of the elite taught Latin and, sometimes, Greek. Some elite schools required students to speak exclusively in Latin.[41]

In Jane Austen's novels, we can find a distinction in the use of Latinate words between high and low status characters.[42]

David Corson,[43] professor at the University of Toronto, claimed that English continues to contain two incompatible vocabularies, one Anglo-Saxon the other Graeco-Latinate. The Anglo-Saxon words are used for the concrete while Greek and Latin words reserved used for more abstract discourse. Graeco-Latinate words are used in higher education and specialist vocabularies

Some English speakers, generally those with better educated parents, learn the Graeco-Latinate lexicon from exposure at home. Those, who come from homes where only concrete Anglo-Saxon words are used, enter school with a real disadvantage. Corson describes this disadvantage as the "lexical bar" and, even, "lexical apartheid." [44]

In order to function at the levels required by higher education one must be able to penetrate the Latinate vocabulary of the academy. Our failure to teach this vocabulary, dis-empowers students and locks them out of the central discourse of our culture. Corson argues that "children's differences in language ability, more than any other observable factor, affect their potential for success in schooling." [45] For example, we know that reading comprehension is closely correlated with vocabulary ability. [46] Indeed, the correlation between vocabulary and comprehension is so high that vocabulary tests are good substitutes for comprehension tests. [47] Psychologist Edgar Dale even argued that "all education is vocabulary development." [48]

You may recall the advertising slogan "people judge you by the words you use" for a vocabulary improvement program called *Verbal Advantage.* [49] This slogan hints at an essential truth; there are well documented vocabulary differences and these differences have social consequences. School and career success are correlated with vocabulary size. [50]

Vocabulary differences are linked to social class and may play a role in perpetuating income inequality. Betty Hart and Todd Risley, of the University of Kansas, found large social class differences in the vocabulary children hear. In their research, they observed 42 families with children for more than two years. The families were from three socioeconomic categories: professional, working class, or welfare. Hart and Risley observed and tape recorded parent-child interactions one hour every month. [51]

Extrapolating from their observations, Hart and Risley found that in a professional family an average child would be exposed to 215,000 words a week. The average child in a working class home would be exposed to 125,000 words. In the family where welfare was the main means of support an average child would be exposed to only 62,000 words per week.

Not surprisingly these differences in exposure were correlated with measures of vocabulary size. Children exposed to more words developed a bigger stock of words. Without educational intervention, these early differences set the stage for lifelong differences in vocabulary.

The Weschler Adult Intelligence Scale is a widely used test of cognitive ability. It has been standardized on large representative samples. Joseph Matarazzo published the percentage of adults between the age of 16 and 65 who could correctly define some of the test's vocabulary items in its 1955 standardization sample. Not surprisingly, everyone could define common physical objects such as a bed or a penny. As words became more abstract, the percentages dropped sharply. Only 65% could define the word "domestic" and only 20% knew the meaning of the word "ominous." The majority did not know the words "calamity," "tranquil," or "fortitude." The word "travesty" was only known to 5% of the sample.[52] As Gottfredson pointed out "none of these words is esoteric; anyone who has attended U.S. high schools or read national newspapers or magazines has surely encountered them. Vocabulary tests gauge the ease with which individuals have routinely caught on to new and more complex concepts they encounter in the general culture." [53]

The difference between the two forms of English is not simply a matter of synonyms. It is not the case that there is a plain-spoken alternative for every hifalutin word used by know-it-all academics. Rather if you speak only Anglo-Saxon English you lack access to powers of analysis given by a more powerful vocabulary.[54] Vocabulary is the single biggest factor predicting reading comprehension. Indeed, vocabulary knowledge is more important than knowledge of grammar for comprehension. [55]

Available evidence suggests that American vocabulary skills have declined over time. We have evidence for this from the WORDSUM test administered as part of the General Social Survey (GSS). The GSS is a national face to face survey conducted annually by the National Opinion Research Center on a large representative sample of the English speaking American public. The WORDSUM is a ten item vocabulary test that is often included in the GSS.[56]

In this test, a person is given a card with a word in capital letters, such as BEAST, and six possible responses. For example, BEAST might be followed by 1. afraid, 2. words, 3. large, 4. animal, 5. separate, and 6, DON'T KNOW. Analysis of people's performance on the WORDSUM suggest that it contains six easy words, which a majority answer correctly, and, four hard words, which are answered correctly only by a minority.[57] At all educational levels only a minority of people interviewed received a perfect score. However, obtaining a perfect score was closely tied to education level. Only 1.4% of those with 0 to 4 years of education received a perfect score, while 36.7% of those with 20 years of education received a perfect score.[58] Reviews of WORDSUM scores adjusted for age and education level show that vocabulary scores have been falling over time.[59]

A variety of explanations have been proposed to explain this decline including a shift to television viewing and away from newspaper reading.[60] Others have argued that the decline is related to textbook simplification. In an effort to make textbooks more accessible and easier to read publishers have used readability algorithms that may have made schoolbooks less challenging. Simplified text books may have created an impoverished linguistic environment for students.[61]

In the account of language given by Soviet psychologist Lev Vygotsky, our internal mental life, that which seems so intimate and private is bound to the larger culture. For humans, language structures the way we think, as children internalize language mental processes become more a kind of self-talk.[62] A number of thinkers have pointed out how our growth in vocabulary is linked to our growth in ideas. Edgar Dale wrote about the "explosive effect" of learning new words "pushing the possessor on to search for new applications. when our words change, we change."[63]

Our academic language has its roots in ancient Greece. The word "academic" itself is Greek in origin referring the estate of Academus that became the place where Plato taught.[64] Classical scholar Bruno Snell noted a vocabulary gulf between the early Greek of Homer and the richer language of the classical period. Over time, the Geeks created a vocabulary that allowed them to express increasingly abstract ideas. The new vocabulary allowed for a shift from egocentric to ideocentric discourse.[65] In a sense, children recapitulate this transformation when they acquire the academic vocabulary, moving from egocentric concerns to a more ideocentric orientation. Acquiring this vocabulary is so important that academic language may be seen as a special language requiring special instruction.[66]

Memory for vocabulary words, then, has an important effect on education and success in life. There is encouraging evidence that we can improve most student's memory for vocabulary words through a process of direct instruction. One promising approach is to teach students the Latin and Greek roots that form the basis for our academic lexicon. In one study, the use of a computerized tutorial on Latin and Greek roots used twice a week for 45 minutes produced substantial improvements in vocabulary for high school students.[67]

Incidental Learning?

This notion of teaching vocabulary especially English language vocabulary flies in the face of the cult of incidental learning. Incidental learning is a real phenomenon. It can be defined as learning without the intention to learn. In memory experiments this refers to situations where a person is exposed to information, but not told in advance that a test will occur. In the world outside the laboratory incidental learning covers the many thing we learn from the environment in an unplanned way. For example, the many words whose meanings we have learned simply from listening to them being used in context.

While it is certainly true that we acquire a large percentage of our vocabulary through inference from context, a large percentage of our academic vocabulary is learned through instruction. The mere existence of incidental learning does not tell us if it is the most appropriate method to teach students the words they need to succeed academically. Indeed, we know that it is more difficult to learn from context from the written word as opposed to the spoken language.[68]

The debate over vocabulary instruction is not limited to learning words in our own language but also over foreign language learning. Language acquisition expert Jan Hulstijn described the terms of the argument. Advocates of incidental learning argue that when learners have to infer meaning from context they expend more mental effort, and consequently better remember information. While, on the other hand, advocates of instructional approaches point out that "context seldom offers enough information for the inferring method to be successfully applied."[69] Hulstijn conducted several experiments comparing incidental to instructional approaches for teaching foreign language vocabularies. He found that retention with incidental learning was "very low indeed."[70]

Hulstijn notes three problems with incidental learning from context. First, the context may not contain enough information to make an inference. Second, there is the real danger that the learner may make an incorrect inference. Finally, students many differ in their ability to infer word meaning.[71]

Incidental learning does have a role. But in foreign language learning, direct teaching of vocabulary and the incidental learning of words from context should be complementary processes.[72]

All this suggests that direct instruction of vocabulary is essential for many students.

David Ausubel's Critique of Incidental Learning

We can think of the debates over vocabulary learning as a prototype for many of the arguments over incidental and more didactic approaches to education. The correct observation that incidental learning takes place becomes the rationale for the claim that most or all teaching should be indirect and grow out of discovery rather than instruction.

This popular belief was perhaps a reaction to the overly regimented approaches to teaching. However, it does not follow that anarchism is the best alternative to authoritarian teaching.

When children learn language from context without special effort we are impressed, but it does not follow that all learning can be effortless and incidental. We rightly react against instruction based on punishment or teaching that is simply boring. This visceral reaction has led some teachers to reject the important drill and practice component of education. The phrase "drill and kill" has been used to dismiss all didactic instruction.

David Ausubel was an influential educational psychologist who died in 2008. While not unsympathetic to many aspects of progressive education he recognized a contradiction between two widely held beliefs. "On the one hand," he wrote, "we minimize the value of drill in educational theory regarding it as rote, mechanical, passive, and old fashioned."[73] On the other hand, educators believe that practice makes perfect. According to Ausubel, this conflict means that when we use drill in the classroom we "do so half-heartedly, apologetically, and in ways that detract from its effectiveness."[74]

Drill is vital to education, it provides practice and feedback. It need not be boring and oppressive. Psychologist Stephen Ray Flora has suggested we need to find ways to "drill and thrill"[75] students.

The Joy of Memory

This "fetish of naturalism and incidental learning"[76] that Ausubel described is related to the anti-memory bias we see in some educators. One under appreciated consequence of this bias may be the disadvantaging of students who excel at memory. It is tragic that students with good memory skills are often discouraged by the school system.

While many educators have disparaged the role of memory in the schools, there are some reform programs that include memorization as a key component. One example of this can be seen in the work of Marva Collins.[77] Collins ran the Westside Preparatory School, a private elementary school that served an impoverished neighborhood in Chicago. She argued that:

> the problem is that some schools cannot strike a balance between "progressive" and "traditional" teaching methods. People wrongly assume that it has to be one or the other. If you teach the basics in a classical curriculum, you can still pay attention to a child's feelings and attitudes. Moreover, it is a mistake to assume that in order to stimulate creativity and critical thinking you must rule out any learning by rote. Memorization is the only way to

teach such things as phonics, grammar, spelling, and multiplication tables.

There is a tendency in education to reject arbitrarily a method of teaching simply because it's old fashioned. The fact is a teacher can combine both progressive and traditional approaches to learning, each enhancing the other. There is no reason why a teacher can't be sensitive to a child's needs and at the same time teach the child subject matter and skills.[78]

Collins' teaching program is called the Great Expectations Initiative. Ronald Ferguson, Senior Lecturer in Education and Public Policy at the Harvard Kennedy School, interviewed Oklahoma teacher Greg Robarts about his experience with the initiative.

Many people who are not familiar with the Great Expectations approach say that it overemphasizes memorization and under emphasizes higher order thinking. Robarts disagrees. He says these functions are compliments, not substitute: memory is the foundation for higher order thinking. He finds that without practice at memorization many children cannot remember a dictated sentence long enough to write it down. After a few weeks of memorizing poetry and other things, he says, the change is remarkable. He thinks that people who dismiss memory work as outmoded are simply uninformed about how children learn, not only because memory supports higher order thinking, but because children can memorize things that are worth knowing. In addition, by reciting what they have memorized, children build up self-confidence and motivation.[79]

Background Knowledge

Many children (and not a few adults) think that the abbreviation AD means After Death. We can all think of examples of someone not knowing a piece of basic information or fundamentally misunderstanding a concept. We are startled when a friend says "Greenwich Village Time" instead of "Greenwich Mean Time." These errors are not simply vocabulary errors. It is not just a matter of having the wrong word; it is that having the wrong word reflects confusion over meaning. The idea that AD means After Death defies logic. If you think that it is Greenwich Village Time, you may have other fundamental misunderstandings about the system of longitude and how time is calculated.

A friend of my daughter once noticed our copy of *Grey's Anatomy*. She was disappointed when she pulled the book off the shelf and discovered it was not about the TV show *Gray's Anatomy*. She was not aware of the existence of the famous book and, thus, did not get the joke in the title of her favorite show. The point is that we need background information to understand the world we live in. Without background information, the world is mysterious. Indeed, lack of knowledge can have far reaching consequences.

The National Science Foundation reported that "Scientific literacy in the United States (and in other countries) is fairly low. Scientific literacy is defined as "knowing basic facts and concepts about science and having an understanding of how science works." [80] Only 11% of American adults can correctly define radiation. [81]

Our cultural prejudice against knowledge often

reflects a profound lack of curiosity. Not knowing something is not a deficit, it is an occasion to learn and we should welcome these opportunities. Psychologist James Weinland wrote that "knowledge creates interest, interest leads to more knowledge, more knowledge to more interest, and so on ad infinitum."[82]

The case for memory is a case for curiosity, for the open mind, and for lifelong learning. The goal is not a mountain of disconnected facts, but information organized into rich knowledge of the world. We can train our memories, we can improve our powers of recall and this is a goal well worth pursuing. A point made so well by Ralph Waldo Emerson, "the Past has a new value every moment to the active mind, through the incessant purification and better method of its memory." [83]

1   Jacoby, S. (2008). *The age of American unreason.* New York: Pantheon Books.

2   Kohn, A. (2000). *The schools our children deserve: moving beyond traditional classrooms and "tougher standards."* Boston: Houghton Mifflin Company.(p. 54).

3   Kohn, A. (2000). *The schools our children deserve : moving beyond traditional classrooms and "tougher standards."* Boston: Houghton Mifflin Company.(p. 122).

4   Berliner, D. C., and Biddle, B. J. (1995). *The manufactured crisis; Myths, fraud, and the attack on America's public schools.* Reading, MA: Addison-Wesley Publishing Company. (pp. 300 -301)

5   Berliner, D. C., and Biddle, B. J. (1995). *The manufactured crisis; Myths, fraud, and the attack on America's public schools.* Reading, MA: Addison-Wesley Publishing Company. (p. 302).

6   Bloom, B. S. (Ed.) (1956). *Taxonomy of educational objectives: The classification of educational goals, by a committee of college and university examiners.* New York: David McKay & Company.

7   Caine, R. N. & Caine, G. (1990). Understanding a brain-based approach to learning and teaching. *Educational Leadership, 48,* 66 - 70.(p. 69)

8   Bloom, B. S. (Ed.) (1956). *Taxonomy of educational*

objectives: The classification of educational goals, by a committee of college and university examiners. New York: David McKay & Company. (p. 18)

9 Hayes-Roth, B. & Walker, C. (1977). *Configural effects in human memory.* Santa Monica, CA: The Rand Corporation.

10 Bernstien, A. & Roberts, M. V. (1958). Computer v. chess-player. *Scientific American, 198,* 96 - 105.

11 Hayes-Roth, B. & Walker, C. (1977). *Configural effects in human memory.* Santa Monica, CA: The Rand Corporation.(p. 1)

12 Gobet, F. & Simon, H. A. (1996). Recall of random and distorted positions: Implications for the theory of expertise. *Memory & Cognition, 24,* 493-503

13 Hayes-Roth, B. & Walker, C. (1979). Configural Effects in Human Memory: The superiority of memory over external information sources as a basis for inference verification. *Cognitive Science, 3,* 119 - 140. (p. 123)

14 Hayes-Roth, B. & Walker, C. (1979). Configural Effects in Human Memory: The superiority of memory over external information sources as a basis for inference verification. *Cognitive Science, 3,* 119 - 140.(p. 139).

15 Wingfield, A. & Byrnes, D. L. (1981). *The psychology of human memory.* New York: Academic Press.

16 Emerson, R. W. (1974). *The portable Emerson.* Van Doren, M. (Ed.). New York: Penguin Books. (p. 272)

17 Stern, L. (1985). *The structures and strategies of human memory.* Homewood, IL: The Dorsey Press.

18 Staszewski, J. J. (1990). Exceptional memory: The influence of practice and knowledge on the development of encoding strategies. In W. Schneider & E. E. Weindert (Eds.), *Interactions among aptitudes, strategies, and knowledge in cognitive performance* (pgs. 252 – 285). New York: Springer-Verlag.

19 Sweller, J. (2009). Human cognitive architecture and constructivism. In Tobias, S. & Duffy, T. M. (Eds.). *Constructivist instruction; Success or failure?* (Pages 127 - 143). New York: Routledge. (p. 131).

20 Jacoby, S. (2008). *The age of American unreason.* New York: Pantheon Books.(p. 17).

21 Gordon, K. (1933). Some records of the memorizing of sonnets. *Journal of Experimental Psychology,16,* 701-708.

22 Wingfield, A. & Byrnes, D. L. (1981). *The psychology of human memory.* New York: Academic Press.

23 Morris, P. E., Gruneber, M. M., Sykes, R. N., & Merrick, A. (1981). Football knowledge and the acquisition of new results. *British Journal of*

Psychology, 72, 479 – 483.

24 James, W. (1899/1958). *Talks to teachers: On psychology; and to students on some of life's ideals.* New York: W. W. Norton & Company. (p. 91).

25 Emerson, R. W. (1974). *The portable Emerson.* Van Doren, M. (Ed.). New York: Penguin Books. (p. 271).

26 Radvansky, G. A. (2011). *Human memory.* Boston; Allyn & Bacon. (p. 3).

27 Ley, P. (1978). Memory for medical information. In M. M. Gruneberg, P. E. Morris, & R. N. Sykes (Eds.). *Practical aspects of memory.* (pp. 120 - 127). London: Academic Press.

28 Weinland, J. D. (1957). *How to improve your memory.* New York: Barnes and Noble, Inc. (p. 18).

29 Kyllonen, P. C., Tirre, W. C., & Christal, R. E. (1991). Knowledge and processing speed as determinants of associative learning. *Journal of Experimental Psychology: General,* 120, 57 -79. (p. 58)

30 Sternberg, R. J. (2009). Forward. In Tobias, S. & Duffy, T. M. (Eds.). *Constructivist instruction; Success or failure?* (Pages x - xi). New York: Routledge. (p. x)

31 Vargas, J. S. (2009). *Behavior analysis for effective teaching.* New York: Routledge.

32 Nation, I.S. P. (2001). *Learning vocabulary in another language.* Cambridge, UK: Cambridge

University Press.

33 Gardner, H. (1991). *The unschooled mind: How children think and how schools should teach.* New York: Basic Books. (1991)

34 Nation, I.S. P. (2001). *Learning vocabulary in another language.* Cambridge, UK: Cambridge University Press.

35 Nation, I.S. P. (2001). *Learning vocabulary in another language.* Cambridge, UK: Cambridge University Press.

36 Nagy, W. E., & Herman, P. A. (1987). Breadth and depth of vocabulary knowledge: Implications for acquisition and instruction. In M. G. McKeown & M. E. Curtis (Eds.). *The nature of vocabulary acquisition.* (pp. 19 - 35). Hillsdale, NJ: Lawrence Erlbaum Associates.

37 Snell, R. (2010). *Read and write Hindi script.* London: Teach Yourself.

38 Ibrahim, R. (2009). The cognitive basis of diglossia in Arabic: Evidence from a repetition priming study within and between languages. *Psychology Research and Behavior Management, 2;* 93 - 105.

39 Corson, D. (1985). *The lexical bar.* Oxford: Pergamon Press.

40 McQuaun, J. & Malless, S. (1998). *Coined by Shakespeare: Words & meanings first penned by the Bard.* Springfield, MA: Merriam-Webster Incorporated.

41 Corson, D. (1985). *The lexical bar.* Oxford:

Pergamon Press.

42 DeForest, M., & Johnson, E. (2001). The density of Latinate words in the speeches of Jane Austen's characters. *Literary and Linguistic Computing, 16,* 389 - 401.

43 Corson, D. (1985). *The lexical bar.* Oxford: Pergamon Press.

44 Corson, D. (1985). *The lexical bar.* Oxford: Pergamon Press. (p. 35)

45 Corson, D. (1985). *The lexical bar.* Oxford: Pergamon Press. (p. 1).

46 Sternberg, R. J. (1987). Most vocabulary is learned from context. In M. G. McKeown & M. E. Curtis (Eds.). *The nature of vocabulary acquisition.* (pp. 89 - 105). Hillsdale, NJ: Lawrence Erlbaum Associates.

47 Chall, J. S. (1987). Two vocabularies for reading: Recognition and meaning. In M. G. McKeown & M. E. Curtis (Eds.). *The nature of vocabulary acquisition* (pp. 7 - 17). Hillsdale, NJ: Lawrence Erlbaum Associates.

48 Dale, E. & O'Rourke, J. (1971). *Techniques of teaching vocabulary.* Palo Alto, CA: Field Educational Publications. (p. 5).

49 Elster, C. H. (2000). *Verbal advantage: 10 Steps to a Powerful Vocabulary.* New York: Random House.

50 Broadley, M. E. (2002).*Your natural gifts: How to recognize and develop them for success and*

self-fulfillment. Marshall, VA: EPM Publications
51 Hart, B. & Risley, T. R. (1995). *Meaningful differences in the every day experiences of young America children.* Baltimore, MD: Paul H. Brooks Publishing Company.
52 Matarazzo, J. D. (1972). *Wechsler's measurement and appraisal of adult intelligence.* (5th edition). New York: Oxford University Press.

53 Gottfredson, L. S. (1997). Why *g* matters: The complexity of everyday life. *Intelligence, 24,* 79 – 132. (p. 95)
54 Corson, D. (1985). *The lexical bar.* Oxford: Pergamon Press.
55 Chall, J. S. (1987). Two vocabularies for reading: Recognition and meaning. In M. G. McKeown & M. E. Curtis (Eds.). *The nature of vocabulary acquisition* (pp. 7 - 17). Hillsdale, NJ: Lawrence Erlbaum Associates.
56 Malhotra,N., Krosnick, J. A., & Haertel, E. (2007). *The psychometric properties of the GSS WORDSUM vocabulary test.* GSS Methodology Report No. 111. Chicago: NORC.

57 Malhotra,N., Krosnick, J. A., & Haertel, E. (2007). *The psychometric properties of the GSS WORDSUM vocabulary test.* GSS Methodology Report No. 111. Chicago: NORC.

58 Glenn, N. D. (1994). Television watching,

newspaper reading, and cohort differences in verbal ability. *Sociology of Education, 67,* 216 - 230.

59 Hayes, D. P., Wolfer, L. T., & Wolfe, M. F. (1996). Schoolbook simplification and its relation to the decline in SAT-Verbal scores. *American Educational Research Journal, 33,* 489 - 508.

60 Glenn, N. D. (1994). Television watching, newspaper reading, and cohort differences in verbal ability. *Sociology of Education, 67,* 216 - 230.

61 Hayes, D. P., Wolfer, L. T., & Wolfe, M. F. (1996). Schoolbook simplification and its relation to the decline in SAT-Verbal scores. *American Educational Research Journal, 33,* 489 - 508.

62 Vygotsky, L. S. (1978). *Mind in society: The development of higher psychological processes.* Cambridge, MA: Harvard University Press.

63 Dale, E. & O'Rourke, J. (1971). *Techniques of teaching vocabulary.* Palo Alto, CA: Field Educational Publications. (p. 9)

64 Asivov, I. (1959). *The words of science: And the history behind them.* Cambridge, MA: The Riverside Press.

65 Snell, B. (1960). *The discovery of mind: The Greek origin of European thought.* New York: Harper & Row.

66 Stotsky, S. (1985). From egocentric to ideocentric discourse: The development of academic language. In J. A. Niles & R. V. Lalik (Eds.). *Issues in literacy:*

A research perspective. (pp. 21 - 29). Rochester, NY: National Reading Conference.

67 Holmes, C. T., & Keffer, R. L. (1995). A computerized method to teach Latin and Greek root words: Effect on verbal SAT scores. *The Journal of Educational Research, 89,* 47 - 50.

68 Nagy, W. E., & Herman, P. A. (1987). Breadth and depth of vocabulary knowledge: Implications for acquisition and instruction. In M. G. McKeown & M. E. Curtis (Eds.). *The nature of vocabulary acquisition.* (pp. 19 - 35). Hillsdale, NJ: Lawrence Erlbaum Associates.

69 Hulstijn, J. H. (1992). Retention of inferred and given word meanings: Experiments in incidental vocabulary learning. In P. J. L. Arnaud & H. Bejoint. *Vocabulary and applied linguistics.* (pp. 113 - 125). Hampshire, UK: Macmillan Academic and Professional. (p. 114)

70 Hulstijn, J. H. (1992). Retention of inferred and given word meanings: Experiments in incidental vocabulary learning. In P. J. L. Arnaud & H. Bejoint. *Vocabulary and applied linguistics.* (pp. 113 - 125). Hampshire, UK: Macmillan Academic and Professional. (p. 122)

71 Hulstijn, J. H. (1992). Retention of inferred and given word meanings: Experiments in incidental vocabulary learning. In P. J. L. Arnaud & H. Bejoint. *Vocabulary and applied linguistics.* (pp. 113 - 125).

Hampshire, UK: Macmillan Academic and Professional.

72 Nation, I.S. P. (2001). *Learning vocabulary in another language.* Cambridge, UK: Cambridge University Press.

73 Ausubel, D. P. (1969). *Readings in school Learning.* New York: Holt, Rinehart, & Winston. (p. 210).

74 Ausubel, D. P. (1969). *Readings in school Learning.* New York: Holt, Rinehart, & Winston. (p. 210)

75 Flora, S. R. (2004). The power of reinforcement. Albany, NY: State University of New York. (p. 7)

76 Ausubel, D. P. (1969). *Readings in school Learning.* New York: Holt, Rinehart, & Winston. (p. 211)

77 Ferguson, R. F. (1998). Teacher's perceptions and expectations and the black white test score gap. In C. Jencks & M. Phillips (Eds.). *The black-white test score gap.* (PP. 273 – 317). Washington, D. C.: Brookings Institute.

78 Collins, M. & Tamarkin, C. (1990). *Marva Collins' way: Returning to excellence in education.* New York: Penguin Putnam, Inc. (p. 132)

79 Ferguson, R. F. (1998). Teacher's perceptions and expectations and the black white test score gap. In C. Jencks & M. Phillips (Eds.). *The black-white test score gap.* (PP. 273 – 317). Washington, D. C.: Brookings Institute. (p. 308)

80 National Science Board (2004). *Science and engineering indicators* National Science

Foundation: Washington, DC. (Chapter 7, p. 15)

81 Miller, J. D. (2004). Public understanding of, and attitudes toward, scientific research: what we know and what we need to know. *Public Understanding of Science, 13*, 273–294

82 Weinland, J. D. (1957). *How to improve your memory.* New York: Barnes and Noble, Inc. (p. 49)

83 Emerson, R. W. (1974). *The portable Emerson.* Van Doren, M. (Ed.). New York: Penguin Books. (p. 272)

Chapter 3

The Science of Memory

Some years ago, I read a chapter in a book by the great polymath Martin Gardner on memorizing numbers. Gardner described a widely used system of converting numbers to consonants. I tried the technique and was impressed with the results. [1] Although I eventually abandoned this technique, and now use the one advocated by memory champion Dominic O'Brien (described in Chapter 7), it was reading Gardner that hooked me on mnemonic systems.

Later, while pursuing my doctorate in education, I came to the scientific study of memory. Reading across several sub-disciplines of psychology, educational, developmental, cognitive, and behavioral, I realized that real progress has been made in our understanding of how memory works and how it can be improved. Throughout this book, I will describe some of these important insights. This will be a departure from some memory improvement books that focus on techniques, but say little about the scientific background. That science of education teaches us that we are much more likely to adopt and apply a new skill if we know why it works.

Defining Memory and Learning

In the broadest sense, memory is the storing of information. Of course, we store information in all kinds of ways: in books, on post it notes, computer hard drives, and so forth. These types of information storage are sometimes described as external memory. Occasionally, I will use examples of external memory for compassion and contrast with human memory. However, since our knowledge of the actual processes of human memory has been increasing, it is often possible to describe memory storage directly in biological terms. Thus, the need for analogies has been reduced. Unlike Plato, who compared memory to a writing on a wax tablet, we can now talk about changes in the structure and organization of neurons.

Memory is closely related to learning. Indeed, memory and learning are dependent upon each other. There can be no learning without memory, and memory without learning is meaningless. Psychologists have struggled to form an adequate definition of learning.[2] Here I will use a definition that I think distills the most important features of our modern understanding. Learning is a change in behavior potential due to experience. While the definition is short, it requires some explanation.

Behavior is anything an animal, including the human animal, does. It is the way an animal acts in the world. Some of our behavior is fixed and hardwired at birth. A baby spider does not learn how to spin her web at her mother's eight knees. A spider is born knowing how to construct its web. We do not have to be taught how to kick in response to the doctor's hammer. Inborn reflexive behaviors are not learned. But some behaviors can be modified by experience. For example, even very simple animals, such as insects, can learn the best route through a maze. [3] This ability to change, this behavioral flexibility, is crucial for our survival in the world. If the environment was static, we would not need to learn, all our behaviors could be passed on through the genes and only improved by natural selection. One advantage of hard wired instinctual behaviors is that we are born able to deploy them without wasting time for learning. Thus, roaches, for example, have evolved a very stable and successful set of instinctual behaviors. No time is wasted in learning new skills: There may be roach motels but there are no roach universities.

However, in unstable environments it is often more adaptive to have behavioral flexibility. That is, the ability to alter behavior in response to changing conditions. Many animals, especially humans, rely heavily on this capacity to learn. Learning about the environment requires the ability to acquire, store, and update information in memory.

Our definition specifies that learning is a change in behavior potential. We know from our own experience that learning does not always change our behavior. You may learn some fact about the world, for example, the metric circumference of the earth is about 40,000 kilometers, but if no one ever asks you about it your behavior remains unchanged. However, your behavior potential has been altered, if asked, you are able to provide the correct answer.

A simple example of learning is Pavlovian conditioning. Most of us are familiar with Pavlov's famous experiment where a dog learned to salivate to a sound. To avoid retelling this too familiar story, and to emphasize that Pavlovian learning is not limited to dogs, I'll describe Pavlovian conditioning in humans.

There is standard laboratory procedure for studying Pavlovian conditioning in people, but it does not involve saliva and the presentation of food (although such experiments, often involving the weighing of dental cotton stuffed in the mouth, have been performed on people). It is called eyeblink conditioning. In this procedure the participant (the word "subject" has fallen out of vogue) wears a set of special glasses that holds one end of a plastic tube close to the eye. The experimenter can send a harmless puff of air through the tubing to the participant's cornea, invoking a reflexive eye blink. We call the eye blink reflex an unconditioned response. It is not learned; it is an inborn response to some environmental stimulus.

If the experimenter plays an electronic tone and it has no effect on the participant, we call the tone a neutral stimulus. However, if the tone is played every time the eye is puffed with air, over time, even in the absence of the air puff, the tone itself will cause the eyes to blink. The participant has learned an association between two events in the environment, the tone and the air puff. An association has been made, and behavior has changed as a result of experience. Somehow, that experience has changed the behavior potential of the nervous system. Some information about the world (the relationship between tone and air puff) is now stored in memory.

An alternative procedure involves conditioning changes in the electrical conductivity of the skin. Skin conductance is measured by passing a small electrical current between two electrodes on the skin. The electrical current is so small that it cannot be felt and poses no danger to the volunteer. Generally the electrodes are attached the palm of one hand or to onto two fingers on the same hand. A surprising or threatening event, or other strong emotional stimulus, causes the conductivity of the skin to increases. In other words, the skin temporarily becomes a better conductor. This reaction is unlearned and automatic and is sometimes called the skin conductance response. It is believed that the conductivity of the skin is controlled by the sweat glands. Sweat, of course, is involved in the regulation of body temperature, but sweat glands also become more active in stressful situations. Most of us of have had the experience of clammy, sweaty hands, associated with high anxiety.[4] By pairing a neutral stimulus, such as a buzzer, with one that provokes distress, such as a mild electric shock, a person can be conditioned to increase skin conductance to sound of the buzzer alone.

While eyeblink and skin conductance conditioning might seem to be useful only for demonstrations in an undergraduate psychology class, they are, in fact, extremely powerful procedures that give us insight into many important human behaviors. For example, a body of research has developed on individual differences in conditioning. It has been discovered that psychopaths, a term used to describe people who are temperamentally antisocial, condition at a much slower rate than non-psychopathic controls. This is significant since there is evidence that some of our ideas about appropriate and inappropriate behaviors are learned through Pavlovian conditioning.[5] Poor eyeblink conditioning in older adults may also be an early symptom of Alzheimer's disease.[6]

We can learn a lot about memory from studying simple forms of learning. More complex forms of learning are built up from the building blocks of simple learning. It is, in fact, possible to construct a hierarchy of learning from the simple to the more complex types.

The two simplest forms of learning, habituation and sensitization, involve the modification of reflexes. As already noted, a reflex is hard wired unlearned response to some event in the environment. For example, an eye blink in response to some irritation to the cornea is a reflex. It is an automatic unlearned adaptive behavior.

In habituation, we learn to reduce the strength of a reflex after repeated exposure to some stimulus. Animals, who are at first frightened of us and flee, may over time become habituated to our presence. The bird, once scared of you, learns to eat from your hand. The first time someone taps you on the shoulder you jump up and your heart races in a classic startle response. But if you are tapped often enough you learn to respond calmly. Your startle response had been habituated.[7]

In sensitization, we increase the strength of a reflex after repeated exposure. Soldiers often become more sensitive to the sound of incoming artillery, not less. This type of sensitization learning is believed to be a major component of post-traumatic stress disorder.[8]

Habituation and sensitization are called non-associative learning, and they stand at the bottom of our learning hierarchy. Associative learning is more complex. There are two types of associative learning: Pavlovian conditioning and operant conditioning. They are called associative because they both involve learning about associations in the world. Or instead of associations we might say relationships or correlations. Associative learning tells us something about relationships in our environment. In Pavlovian conditioning we learn that some stimulus that previously had no effect on our behavior actually predicts some outcome that is important to us, and we learn to respond to that stimulus. If the sound of the buzzer predicts an irritant to the eye, it makes sense to blink in response to the buzzer.

In operant conditioning, we learn to modify our behavior in response to its consequences. If our behavior has reinforcing consequences then we are more likely to engage in that behavior in the future. If the consequence of our behavior is punishing than we are less likely to behave in the same way.

At the top of the learning hierarchy are more complex forms of learning such as observational learning and rule governed behaviors. In observational learning we learn, not from our own direct experience, but from watching someone else's actions. By observing the consequences of that person's actions, we change our own behavior. Rule governed behavior is learning through language. A rule is a verbal description of the predictive relationship between events. We can be told that a certain action is likely to have some consequence and modify our behavior accordingly.

Behavioral and Cognitive Psychology

Psychology has long been divided into two general approaches behaviorism and cognitivism. Behaviorism grew out of frustration with subjective accounts of mental processes and drew the conclusion that internal mental states could not be the subject of scientific investigation. Inferences could only be drawn about the relationships between observable changes in the environment and observable changes in behavior. Regularities in these relationships could then be formulated as scientific laws.

Generally, behavioral psychologists have avoided the word "memory," and preferred to speak in terms of "remembering" and "verbal learning." This reluctance to use a widely understood concept has led to some remarkable verbal somersaults. For example, in the words of one behaviorist "the study of remembering is concerned with how an organism's present behavior can be occasioned by past events, as when a delay is imposed between stimulus and response."[9]

Cognitive psychologists, on the other hand, have not shied away from inferring internal mental processes and structures and memory is defined as "the retention of experience dependent internal representations over time."[10]

In recent years, cognitive psychology has held the upper hand, and undergraduate psychology textbooks often speak of a cognitive revolution occurring in the

1960s. However, claims of a revolution in psychology seem a bridge too far. The discoveries of behavioral psychology have not been eclipsed or abandoned, and it may be more accurate to describe cognitive psychology as broadening of perspective rather than as a revolution. The principles of classical and operant conditioning continue to explain a wide range of behavior, and the behaviorists were right to remind us that our inferences about psychological processes must rely on observations of behavior. On the other hand, the strictures placed on inference by some behaviorists were too extreme. Here we would do well to follow the lead of the great cognitive -behavioral psychologist Edward Chace Tolman.

Tolman believed that, like in other sciences, it is legitimate for psychologists to infer the existence of hidden variables and structures if these variables improve our ability to make predictions. For example, the existence of the atom is, ultimately, an inference, since we cannot observe one directly. Yet, it is impossible to imagine modern chemistry without atoms. Knowing the properties of the invisible atoms allows chemists to make accurate predictions about how different elements will combine.

An example, of such an inference in psychology, is Tolman's evidence for the existence of latent learning and cognitive maps in rats.[11]

In the basic maze learning experiment, a hungry rat is placed into a maze. But wait a second! How do we know the rat is hungry? Isn't hunger a description of an internal mental state? Aren't we anthropomorphizing rats? All good questions; to keep within the behaviorist approach we need to operationalize hunger. By operationalize, I mean defined in terms of some kind of measurement. In this case, we might define a rat as hungry if it has not been fed for some fixed number of hours.

The maze has many blind alleys, but after many wrong turns the rat finally finds its way to its goal, a food box. The experimenter counts the number of wrong turns taken by the rat and records the time it takes the rat to find the food.

The experiment is repeated every 24 hours and over time the rat's performance improves. It makes fewer errors and takes less time to find the food.

There are a number of ways to interpret the rat's maze learning. Most of them involved some variation of Edward Thorndike's law of effect: behaviors that lead to satisfying results tend to be strengthened.[12] So if running the maze correctly leads to food, then the route that leads to this satisfying result will strengthened. These ideas were stated more precisely by B. F. Skinner, who described how the consequences of behavior affected the probability the behavior would recur. What we would like to know is if this model can adequately describe learning without recourse to some kind of description of mental structures? Tolman demonstrated that it could not.

For example, in one experiment, conducted by Tolman's student, Hugh Blodgett, a group of rats was allowed to explore the maze for six days. For those six days there was no food in the food box, and the rats were fed only after they were returned to their home cages. Over those six days there was no improvement in the rats performance.

On the seventh day and all subsequent days, food was placed in the food box. On day 8, these rats demonstrated an "astounding" drop in the number of wrong turns made and time to complete the maze.[13] Once the food was introduced these rats improved their performance much faster than rats in the standard experiment. There seemed to be only one possible explanation, even though there was no reward for maze exploration over the first six days the rats had been learning the maze. They were engaged in latent learning, learning that must have taken place even though it occurred without reinforcement and with no initial effect on behavior. Tolman, in subsequent experiments, demonstrated that the rats must have been building up a cognitive map, a mental representation of the maze.

You can get a sense of latent learning and cognitive maps by trying to answer this question: how many windows does your home or apartment have? Most of us will not immediately know the answer to this question. But, we are likely to use a similar technique to find the answer, we will visualize home and count the windows. We find the answer in the cognitive map stored in our head. Tolman's great contribution was to recognize the strength of the behaviorist program, but also to transcend it in the face of compelling evidence.

We can extend Toman's project when we realize that behavioral observation is not the only source of data that allows us to make reasonable inferences about the structure of human cognition, information about brain processes, structures, and physiology also may be considered. This is particularly true in the case of memory.

Contrary to the strict behaviorist view, it makes sense to speak of memory. We need not put the word "memory" in quotation marks as some behaviorists have.[14] We can infer from the behavioral evidence that information is stored in the nervous system. In addition, by experiment and observation we have learned a great deal about how this storage system works. We now also know something of the underlying biological processes of the brain's information storage. When we speak with confidence of a computer's memory it is because we have good knowledge of the structures that store information. This is not surprising since we created these machines. As we discover the functional and structural basis for the brain's information storage, we should be equally free to describe it as memory. Just as we might define a computer's memory as some configuration of fields on a magnetic medium, we can define a specific human memory as a configuration of brain neurons.[15]

Having made these criticisms of behaviorism, we must recognize that behavioral psychologists continue to make discoveries of immense theoretical and practical value and the consequence for ignoring their work is ignorance.

Is the Mind Absorbent?

In a famous book, Maria Montessori described children as having an absorbent mind.[16] In a similar vein, adults often describe children as being like "little sponges" soaking up information from the environment. Unfortunately, the reality is somewhat more complicated. It would be more correct to say that we are born with a bias towards learning certain types of information. We know that many animals have these biases. A good example of this is the phenomenon is taste aversion learning, sometimes called the Garcia Effect.

To this day, I hate canned creamed corn. Writing about it, indeed, just thinking about it, makes me nauseous. Most of us have some kind of food aversion. We can conjure up the image of some food that we can't stand. Frequently we can recall a specific incident where we became ill eating that food. These food aversions represent a special kind of learning.

John Garcia, a psychologist at the University of California, discovered food aversion learning while investigating the effects of radiation on rats. A non-lethal dose of radiation can cause nausea in a rat. Garcia found that if he presented a rat with saccharine flavored water and exposed it to the nausea inducing radiation, the rat developed an aversion to the saccharine flavor. In some respects, this resembled typical Pavlovian conditioning; a neutral stimulus, the flavor, was paired with an unconditioned stimulus, the radiation. The flavor then became a conditioned stimulus that brought about a conditioned response, nausea. However, there were two crucial differences. While ordinary Pavlovian conditioning took multiple pairings, food aversion conditioning often required a single pairing of food and nausea. Second, Garcia discovered that he could not induce food aversion for unflavored water.

For omnivorous animals such as rats and humans,

it is highly adaptive to be able to learn quickly that some potential food source is poisonous. This "memory for poison," as Garcia called it, is a case of an evolved, inherited, bias to learn certain types of information.[7]

Another example of this kind of prepared learning is our susceptibility to phobias. It is not coincidental that some phobias, such as fear of snakes and spiders, are more common than others. We seem prepared to develop phobias to dangers that plagued our ancestors.

It is easy to see why food aversion learning or phobia preparedness was adaptive for our ancestors and why it would have been passed on to us by natural selection. It seems reasonable that there might be other types of learning for which the human brain might have evolved a talent. Language is, perhaps, the clearest example of this.

For humans, culture is our primary strategy for adapting to the environment and culture rests on our linguistic skills. There is strong evidence that we are biologically programmed to learn language. Children exhibit strong imitative behaviors in speech production and adults seem primed to reinforce correct expression. If a normal child is raised in a language rich environment, the child will learn the language. Which language we learn is a function of the linguistic environment in which we are reared, but, regardless of the specific language, the vast majority of people become competent speakers of their native tongue.

Adults are naturally impressed by the explosion of language skills in young children, but we commit an error if we assume that biological preparation for language learning is the model for all learning. Reading and writing are different from speech. Reading is a cultural invention of relatively recent origin. While we evolved to speak we did not evolve to read and many individuals find learning to read difficult. A similar story can be told about many of the subjects we value. We are born with some ability to understand quantification, but our brains did not evolve to do higher mathematics. Humans have a naïve set of beliefs about physics that have to be unlearned to comprehend modern physics. Thus, we are faced with the reality that much of what we need to learn does not come easily. Learning is hard work and for many academic subjects the model of the absorbent mind is misleading.

Take, for example, memorizing the alphabet. This is a difficult learning task, involving remembering a series of 26 letters in a completely arbitrary order. Most of us master this as children, but is it because we had an absorbent mind as children, now lost to us in adulthood? No. We mastered the alphabet by using mnemonic strategies. We organized the alphabet into three chunks treating multiple elements single units. For children, and even for many adults, the alphabet is [(ab — cd) (ef — g)] [(hi — jk)] [(lmno — p)] [(qrs — tuv) (wxyz)]. Kids learn the alphabet as a mnemonic rhyme and only later learn the meaning of individual components.[18] I am sure that I was not the only child who thought there was a letter named "elemeno."

This, however, need not be cause for despair. It may be possible, in many cases, to bootstrap secondary biological learning unto more basic skills. Later, we will see that we can use the evolved human ability for spatial memory as a basis for a mnemonic system called the method of loci.

Memory and Age

There is a general decline in memory with age that seems to affect all of us, this is called benign senescent forgetting and is not considered pathological. [19] Naturally, we find this forgetting disconcerting. Fortunately, however, there is evidence we can reduce the effects of benign senescent forgetting. We know environmental factors must a role in memory ability because there are differences between generations in performance on memory tests. Standard scores for psychological tests are set by administering them to large representative samples of the general population. When tests are restandardized we can compare changes in test performance across generations. For example, one study found that 61 — 75 years olds tested in 2007, performed better than 61 — 75 year olds tested in 1985.[20] The improvements were substantial and must have some environmental cause since the human genome could not have substantially changed in the intervening decades.

The fact that environmental factors must affect memory is heartening news because it suggests that memory improvement is possible. A subject I'll return to in the next chapter.

How Memory is Organized

Before we can move forward in our understanding of memory we must know something of its structure. We have all heard of short term and long term memory. Unfortunately, these concepts are often misunderstood and misapplied. At this juncture, it would be useful to give a careful description of the memory system by giving an account of how information passes from the outside world into the storage vaults of our brain. Here I will describe three types of memory: sensory memory, working memory (what most people call short term memory), and long term memory.

Shorter than Short Term Memory

The camera's flash lasts for a fraction of a second, yet we continue to see it after the picture is taken. This our common experience is called after image. What we often fail to consider is that the afterimage is a kind of memory; it is the persistence of information in the nervous system.

At any given instant our nervous system is flooded with information. A tsunami of data washes over our sensory system. Photons of light reflect off of objects and onto the retinas of our eyes where photoreceptors transform light into the neuron firings.

The texture of our clothes and the weight of the book in our hands stimulate tactile neurons in our skin. Chemicals in the air cause olfactory cells in our nose to react. Proprioceptors give us information about the position of our limbs in space. The vestibular system of the inner ear provides us with information about balance. We are unaware of most the information flooding into our brains. Much of the information that passes into our nervous system persists for a tiny fraction of a second and then is replaced by new information. That very brief persistence is called sensory memory. It is also called preattentive memory, because while it briefly persists in our nervous system we are largely unaware of it. Generally, this preattentive information exists for a brief instant (from about .25 seconds to 2 seconds) before it new sensory inputs overwrites it.

Only a small fraction of the information that enters our nervous system will come to our conscious awareness. The information we are aware of is said to be in working memory. Working memory is a system that allows us to keep information before our conscious awareness. [21] Short term memory and working memory are similar but not identical concepts. Short term memory is the temporary storage for information that is processed by working memory. Working memory refers to the holding and processing of information before our consciousness awareness. [22] Thus, short term memory can be thought of as a component of working memory. In this book, I will use both terms. Generally, when I want to emphasize storage I will write short term memory. When I want to emphasize the conscious processing of information, I will use working memory.

Two versions of a standard memory test demonstrate the storage and the processing aspects of working memory: forward digit span and reverse digit span.

The forward digit span tests an individual's ability to remember a string of digits. It is a test of capacity, the more digits you can recall the greater your short term memory.

In a the reverse digit span, a test of processing, an individual is read a string of numbers and asked to repeat them in reverse order. As you are likely to guess, for most people reverse digit span is much more difficult than forward digit span. Performance on the reverse digit span correlates with IQ. Performance on the forward digit span does not.

The capacity of short term memory is quite small, usually described as the ability to hold a string of seven digits.[23] Another way to measure the limits of short term memory is pronunciation time. Your short term memory is limited to any list that you are able to pronounce, either vocally or subvocally, in one and a half seconds.[24] In English, we are able to pronounce seven digits within this second and a half time limit. This raises an interesting question. Since numbers are pronounced differently in different languages, does language affect the number of digits a person can hold in short term memory?

Welsh is a Celtic language spoken by more than 600,000 people in Wales. In Welsh, the digits zero to nine are: *dim, un, dau, tri, pedwar, pump, chwech, saith, wyth, naw*. Researchers asked students who spoke both English and Welsh to try reading digits in as fast as possible in both languages. All students, even those who were more fluent in Welsh, were able to pronounce the English digits faster. When tested on forward digit span, the students were able to hold more English digits than Welsh digits in short term memory.[25]

Non-psychologist often misuse and misunderstand the phrase short term memory. Recently, I heard a speaker claim he had terrible short term memory because he could not recall the name of someone he met last year. This was certainly a memory failure, but it was not a failure of short term memory, it was a failure of long term memory. Working memory and short term memory refer only to the temporary storage and processing of information that is before your immediate awareness. If you learned a fact, then thought about something else and were able to recall it once again then the information was in long term memory. Even if you forgot it in a week or a day or an hour that information was in long term memory. Information is only in short term memory when you are aware of it.

As our discussion implies long term memory holds information for longer periods of time, and long term memory is what most of us are interested in when we talk about memory improvement. We want to store information and be able to recover it in the appropriate situations.

As it turns out, long term memory is not a single thing. A distinction has to be made between declarative memory and procedural memory.

Procedural memory is remembering how to do something. How to ride a bicycle, drive a car, juggle, or execute a dance step are all examples of procedural memory. Procedural memory is our memory for skills. Sometimes this is mistakenly labeled "muscle memory," but, of course, memory for executing behaviors resides in the nervous system, not in the muscle.

Declarative memory is the memory of information. Declarative memory can be further divided into episodic memory and semantic memory. Episodic memory is your memory of your personal experience. For example, memory of your high school graduation or first kiss. Semantic memory is your memory for facts, independent of direct experience. Knowing that Columbus is the capitol of Ohio is an example of semantic memory.

There is an interesting relationship between declarative and procedural memory in that many procedural skills are first learned declaratively. When we learn to drive a car, we initially learn a set of instructions — turn the key, then put the foot on the break when shifting into drive, and so on. Later as we become skilled drivers; we do these tasks automatically without thinking about them. Indeed these skills often become so automatic we have trouble describing them. This may explain why expert performers are not always the best teachers; they may lack the declarative vocabulary to describe their procedural mastery.

Pioneering psychologist Donald Hebb suggested an explanation for the underlying differences between short term and long term memory. Hebb hypothesized that in short term memory information is stored in a temporary pattern of nerve cell activation that involved no structural change, while information in long term memory involved some kind of relatively permanent transformation in the structure of neurons or the connections between them. [26] The process of passing information from short term to long term memory, we might also say the process of changing activation patterns into structural patterns, is called consolidation. The actual structural configuration that holds the information is called the memory trace or engram.

Another definition of learning might be the experience driven reorganization of neural pathways. [27] This does not contradict our earlier definition; it merely restates in terms of the underlying neural processes. Learning is a process of brain reorganization. The memory trace is the structural result of that reorganization.

We have learned something about the brain structures involved in memory from the experience of neurosurgery patient named Henry Molaison. Until his death in 2008, Molaison was known to the larger world only by his initials: HM.

From childhood, HM suffered from severe life threatening epilepsy. In a heroic attempt to control his seizures, neurosurgeon William Beecher Scoville, located and removed the areas thought to be the epileptic focal points. The small area of brain tissue removed included structures called the hippocampus. Like many anatomical terms "hippocampus" suggest some imagined similarity. The word means, and the brain structure is said to resemble, a sea horse. Each brain hemisphere has its own hippocampus located at the lower border of the cerebral cortex towards the midline. Scoville removed both the left and right hippocampus and some surrounding tissue from HM's brain.

The surgery succeeded in reducing HM's seizures, but it soon became apparent that it also caused strange pattern of memory loss. HM lost the ability to form new longterm declarative memories. While he could learn new motor skills, and scored above average on an IQ test he was unable to store new facts or events in memory.[28] If you met HM, left the room and returned in a few minutes, he would have no recollection of the first meeting. Every time you met him it would be, for him, the first time.

HM's experience challenged a then popular view that memory could not be localized to any particular structure. Psychologist Karl Lashley, working with rats and monkeys, systematically destroyed areas of their brains and then tested the effects of these ablations on their memory. He found that while the amount of brain tissue destroyed had an effect on the animal's memory, the location of the damage did not. Thus, he concluded that there was no one area where memories were stored. The case of HM forced a refinement of this view. The surgery did not disrupt HM's existing memories, so they could not be said to be stored in the hippocampus. However, the removal of the hippocampus did prevent the consolidation of new long term memories. Thus, there was, at least one, specific brain location critical to the memory process.

Several other cases of hippocampal damage have been reported in the clinical literature that mirror HM's experience. For example, a patient, known by the initials RB, experienced damage to both the right and left hippocampus after heart by-pass surgery. While the tissue destroyed in HM's case included tissue outside the hippocampus. RB's lesions were more limited to the hippocampus. Since his symptoms were similar to those experienced by HM it was reasonable conclude that the hippocampus plays an essential role in the consolidation of declarative information into the long term memory.[29] More recent work has shown that, even in early stages, people with Alzheimer's disease often have a smaller hippocampus.[30]

Brain imaging studies show that the size and structure of the hippocampus changes with learning. London cabdrivers are required to have a detailed knowledge of 25,000 streets and must pass a difficult exam demonstrating this knowledge before being issued taxi license. It takes two to four years of intensive training to master this information. London bus drivers have very similar working conditions to the Taxi drivers, but they are not required to have the same detailed knowledge of the city's layout. When taxi drivers were compared to bus drivers matched for age, gender, education, and IQ, the two groups differed in the distribution of gray matter volume in the hippocampus — the cabbies had more.[31] This research marks some of the clearest evidence that differences in knowledge are associated with structural differences between people's brains.

Information must, some how, be processed by the hippocampus before it can be consolidated into long term memory. Consolidation can be defined as the stabilization of the memory trace.[32] Donald Hebb had proposed that short term memory traces were stored as a pattern of activity in nerve cell firings that soon fade away.[33] In order, for information to enter long term storage it must be stabilized into a relatively permanent structural change in a network of neurons.

Not all memories are affected by hippocampal damage. HM did show improvement of motor skills over time. For example, his ping pong game improved and, with practice, he became better at mirror tracing, a task where one traces a geometric shape while watching the reflection in a mirror. Yet, he could not remember any of his previous practice. In addition, his ability for simple kinds of learning, sensitization, habituation, and Pavlovian conditioning, was unaffected.[34] Thus, it is possible to distinguish between hippocampal dependent memory and hippocampal independent memory.[35] Here we have an example where psychologically distinguishable forms of memory, declarative and procedural, can be associated with different brain structures.

It may be that the hippocampus acts as temporary memory store and that the information is either discarded or moved to some other brain region. Some researchers have purposed that the hippocampus projects and replays information onto neural networks in the brain's neocortex. This replaying may occur during sleep and could be the explanation for our dreams.[36]

The Cycle of Memory

Memory might be described as having a four stage life cycle: acquisition, consolidation, retrieval, and extinction. The memory is born with its acquisition. The memory may die at that point and or it may be consolidated into long term storage. Retrieval refers to accessing the stored memory. Extinction is the death of memory, the withering away of the physical memory trace.[37]

Note that problems can occur at any point in this life cycle. We could fail to acquire information. We could acquire information but fail to consolidate it into our long term memory. The information could be in long term memory, but we might not be able to retrieve it. Finally, the information might simply decay and become extinct.

The Memory Trace

Memory involves physical changes in the brain. Information is a kind of translatable pattern. Edgar Allen Poe's poem, *The Raven*, was written in 1845. Since the time Poe took pen to paper it has been stored in a variety of formats, in the pre-computer age, generally as printed words on a page. A book of poetry may sit on your shelf for decades, but once opened to this particular poem, you can translate the pattern of letters on the page back into a spoken poem.

The Raven has, of course, been stored in many other ways. In 1954, the actor Sir Basil Rathbone made a recording of the poem on a vinyl record, Poe's words being translated into grooves on the record's plastic. Of course, you can now buy Rathbone's rendition on a CD, the pattern translated into tiny pits on the disc that can be read by a laser. Or you can download an mp3 file that stores the information as a pattern in a magnetized medium. These are all forms of memory, information storage.

Fundamentally, human memory is no different,

information must be stored in some physical pattern of the brain that can be reactivated when it is needed.

When we type into a word processor, we think we are communicating in English with the machine. The machine responds to us in English. For example, it notes our spelling errors with a red underline and suggests correctly spelled alternatives. But our computer thinks in a different language, a binary code of ones and zeros. Our inputs are translated into the code. For example, when you depress the key labeled 'a' the computer receives a code of 01100001. This, however, is slightly misleading because the binary value of 01100001 is a pattern of discrete charge states in the computer memory, 1 means a charge, 0 means no charge. Thus, the complete works of Shakespeare, can and has been stored as a very long pattern of charges and no charges that the computer can transform back into the Bard's words.

So your computer does not speak English, what is more surprising is neither does your brain. All information taken in and processed by our brain is encoded in some, still as yet undeciphered, neural code. Our memories are stored as physical patterns in our brain, called memory traces, and only recently have we begun to understand the structure of these traces.

Our memories are consolidated in the changed activity of neurons and in the changed structure of the synaptic connections between neurons. Great progress has been made in our understanding of these processes, although many of the details of the system remain to be worked out.

Looking at the Brain

If memories are stored in the brain there must be some kind of physical change. However, scientific exploration of the brain proved to be extremely difficult. The billions of cells of the brain are packed tightly and initially it was difficult even to see them under a microscope. Even as microscopic techniques improved, early investigators could not see changes associated with learning or even with psychiatric diseases.

The lack of evidence was seized upon by Sigmund Freud as evidence that most mental illness was psychogenic in origin. Freud and his followers asserted that diseases such as schizophrenia and autism were caused by psycho-social factors and could be treated only through psychoanalytic talk therapy.

But even in Freud's time there was evidence for what was called the "anatomical doctrine," the hypotheses that many mental illnesses were organic diseases of the brain. The most persuasive example, at the time, was Alois Alzheimer's discovery of plagues and tangles in the brain of a dementia patient.[38]

The Hunt for the Memory Trace

We do not have enough appreciation for the role of wrong ideas in science. In retrospect, wrong ideas seem misguided or even crazy. Yet, science advances by testing hypotheses and, occasionally, a crazy idea turns out to be true. The exploration of a wrong idea can often be instructive. Even if a wild supposition turns out to be wrong, we frequently gain insights from the testing the hypothesis.

For example, in 19th century America, phrenology, the belief that we could deduce an individual's character from the shape of the skull, was a popular and influential belief. Its supporters included poet Walt Whitman and, the great American educator, Horace Mann. Today we regard phrenology as a ridiculous pseudoscience. Yet, phrenologists, were largely correct in their belief that the brain was a modular organ with localized function, and some phrenologists, such as Franz Gall, made real contributions to the study of brain anatomy.

So with the story of James V. McConnell, in retrospect his work has been ridiculed, yet had he been right, he might have won the Nobel prize. Through his work with flatworms McConnell thought he had discovered the memory trace.

Planaria, are tiny flatworms, each about a centimeter in length, that have two very interesting characteristics; first, they possess a tiny brain, sometimes described as the simplest brain in the animal kingdom, although several other animals might vie for this distinction. Second, planaria have remarkable powers of regeneration. If you cut a flatworm in half down the middle the two halves will grow into separate individuals. If you cut one across the middle into a head and a tail, both halves will also grow into two separate individuals.

McConnell's first experiment was to see if flatworms could learn. He used a very simple classical conditioning procedure. He exposed the worms to light while giving them an electric shock. The shock caused the worms to contract. After pairing the shock and the light a number of times, McConnell's worms would contract to the light even in the absence of the shock. This was a case of classical Pavlovian conditioning. The planaria had learned an association.

In his next experiment, he first conditioned the worms to contract to light. He then cut the worms in half to see if the regenerated planaria would retain the conditioned response. They did.

In another experiment, the one that was to make him famous, he took advantage of the fact that planaria are carnivorous. First, he conditioned a group of worms, then he ground them up and fed them to other the flatworms who had not been conditioned. He found that these cannibals, even thought they had never been taught the association between light and shock, learned to contract in response to the light, faster than planaria that had not eaten schooled planaria. McConnell labeled this phenomenon the "cannibalistic transfer of training."[39]

A clear implication of this research was that if you could understand what chemicals were being transferred you would know the molecular basis of memory. One strong candidate for the memory molecule was ribonucleic acid, better known as RNA. RNA plays a role in genetic processes. It carries instructions from the genes in the cell's nucleus that specify the structure and function of proteins. Thus, RNA was known to be an information bearing molecule. It seemed like a plausible storage mechanism for memory.

McConnell's research created a sensation, and he was not shy about communicating directly with the public. The implication that people might be able to learn complicated academic subjects by simply taking a pill was greeted with enthusiasm.[40] The promise of memory transfer inspired Curt Siodmack, author of the novel *Donovan's Brain* and the screenplay for the *Wolf Man*, to write a science fiction novel, *Hauser's Memory*. In this book a Jewish researcher, in order to uncover information vital for national security, injects himself with RNA extracted from the brain of a Nazi scientist.

McConnell was ultimately vindicated in his claim that planaria possess memory and could learn. But his memory transfer work did not stand. Efforts to replicate it by other research teams failed, and many confounding variables that McConnell had failed to control were identified.[41] McConnell's continued to be an active psychologist writing a widely used introductory textbook. His work on human behavior came to the attention of Unabomber Ted Kaczynski, and McConnell and one his graduate students were seriously injured by a mail bomb.[42]

Evidence of Plasticity

While the memory-RNA hypothesis was a failure, other approaches did begin to clarify the physical mechanisms of memory.

One fundamental question that needed resolving was over the nature of the memory trace, was it dynamic or static? A dynamic trace is one that depends on the continued action of the neurons. We could think of this as the way a plucked string on an instrument continues to make a sound as long as it vibrates. A static trace would involve some kind of physical change in the neurons or the connections between neurons. One piece of evidence for the dynamic trace was the existence of brain waves.

Brain waves, which can be detected by sensitive electrodes placed on the skull, represent the summed electrical activity of neurons, and they are known to change in frequency with different types of mental activity. For example, different levels of sleep will have different brain wave patterns. [43] Perhaps, memories were being stored in a dynamic pattern of bioelectric activity.

In the 1950s, Neurophysiologist Ralph Gerard conceived of an experiment to answer this question. Using hamsters as experimental subjects, he discovered three techniques that would stop all electrical activity in the brain. These techniques were electrical shock, hypoxia (depriving the animal of oxygen for a few minutes), or cooling the animal to 40 degrees Fahrenheit. Hamsters hibernate at that temperature and brain wave activity is suppressed to zero.[44]

The experiment was simple, train the hamsters to run a maze, suppress their brain activity and see if they could still run the maze. Gerard summarized his results in two words, "they remembered!" Thus, he concluded the memory trace must be static.[45]

But not so fast, the picture turned out to be more complicated. It was known that electrical shocks in humans did disrupt memory for information learned shortly before the shock. In addition, some animal researchers reported instances where memory was disrupted by lower temperature. This included humans who reported memory disruption when exposed to extreme cold. Subsequent experiments showed that time between learning and the suppression of brain activity was a critical variable. The longer the information was stored, the more resistant it became to disruption. This was further evidence of a difference between short term and long term memory. This suggested that short term memories might be held dynamically, while long term memories might be stored statically. However, we will see, when we examine Kandel's work, that the differences between short term and long term memory are not rooted in the difference between dynamic and static storage.

The Brains of Rats

As techniques for examining neurons improved direct evidence emerged that learning produced observable changes in the physical structure of the brain. Some of this evidence emerged from what became known as enrichment studies. This line of research entailed comparing the brains of rats raised in the standard laboratory environment with those raised in an enriched environment.

This research was set in motion by the analysis of the brain chemistry of rats. Scientists at Berkeley has discovered that there was a relationship between the levels of the chemical acetylcholinesterase and the performance of rats in a variety of problem solving tests. Acetylcholinesterase is an enzyme that is released in response to the release of the neurotransmitter acetylcholine. The researchers found that the better problems solvers had more acetylcholinesterase in their brains.

Now, it was possible that the smarter rats simply had more of this chemical. But, in the course of their research they found that there was a relationship between the levels of training and the level of acetylcholinesterase. Trained rats had more than untrained rats. Rats who had been trained in more difficult problems than those who were trained in less demanding tasks. Learning itself was changing the chemistry of the rats' brains.[46]

Training the rats in the all the tests was time consuming, so the researchers hit upon a simpler procedure. Raise some rats in an enriched environment with many opportunities for informal learning and raise the other rats in standard lab cages. Rats of the same sex would be randomly assigned to one of the two conditions.

The enriched environment was a large cage with 10 to 12 other rats. The cage included a variety of objects with which the rats could interact. These objects were frequently changed.[47]

Rats raised in the enriched environment had more acetylcholinesterase, greater brain weight, increased sized of neuron cell bodies, and increased number of synapses. While initially greeted with skepticism, these results were replicated other researchers and became part of accepted science.[48]

The fact that physical changes in the structure and size neurons were associated with environmental differences, pointed to a plausible explanation of memory storage, use-dependent plasticity. Neurons were changing in response to the demands placed on them.

A biological tissue is plastic if it changes in structure or function in response to some demand. We may think of our bones as being inert; we remember the lifeless, stone like, skeleton hanging in the science classroom. Appearances are deceiving and, in life, bones are a plastic tissue, reshaped by environmental demands. They will thicken and strengthen in response to exercise and thin and weaken with inactivity. We have a detailed understanding of the underlying forces that shape and reshape bones, the balance in activity between bone building cells and cells that break down bones. The plasticity of neurons in response to environmental inputs has been demonstrated. The structure of the memory trace is found in this plasticity.

The most significant progress towards discovering the memory trace was made by neuroscientist Eric Kandel. Kandel used an approach that was, in some respects, similar to McConnell's work with flatworms. First, Kandel reasoned that it made sense to study learning in a very simple organism. Instead of planaria, Kandel chose Aplaysia, a mollusk also called the sea slug or the sea hare, because it posses two curled tentacles that are said to resemble rabbit ears.[49]

Like the flatworm, the sea slug has a very simple nervous system. However, slugs have one advantage over planaria. They have large neurons that can be easily isolated and studied. In addition, sea slugs are capable of simple learned behaviors.

As we have noted the simplest learned behaviors

are experience based modifications of reflexes, called habituation and sensitization. Sea Slugs have a gill withdrawal reflex. Normally its fragile gill, a breathing organ, extends into the environment. But the sea slug will withdraw its gill into its body when touched, a straightforward gill protection reflex.

Kendal found that he could modify the gill withdrawal reflex, either reducing its intensity (habituation) or increasing it (sensitization). Since he could isolate the specific neurons involved in the reflex, he was able to observe how they changed. He had located a memory trace.

So what is the memory trace? It appears that there is more than one mechanism at work. One that seems particularly important is the long term potentiation of neurons.

Some Background on Neurons

You undoubtedly know that the neuron is the fundamental cell of the nervous system, and that neurons relate to each other through a synapse.

The synapse is the name given to the interface between two neurons. Neurons do not touch each other; they are separated by a small gap called the synaptic cleft. In order to communicate one neuron sends a chemical messenger, called a neurotransmitter across the cleft, where it binds with a receptor. Messages move in only one direction so at any synapse one neuron is always the sender, called the presynaptic neuron, and the other, called the post-synaptic neuron, is always the receiver.

Common neurotransmitters include serotonin,

dopamine, and acetlycholine, although there are many others. Many psychiatric medications work by affecting the brain's levels of neurotransmitters. For example, Prozac and Paxil belong to a class of drugs called SSRIs, selective serotonin re-uptake inhibitors. SSRIs increase the level of the neurotransmitter serotonin between neurons.

When the neurotransmitter attaches to the receptor of the post-synaptic neuron it increases the probability that the post-synaptic neuron will fire and carry a message on to other neurons. However, in order for the post-synaptic neuron to fire it must reach a certain threshold of stimulation.

Our brain is a fantastically complicated network of neurons. There is controversy about how many neurons are contained in the brain. Some estimates exceed a trillion.[50] Most textbooks claim that the brain has 100 billion neurons.[51] Given how difficult it is to count such a large number of minute objects, can we have any confidence in these estimates?

A technique developed by Suzana Herculano-Houzel and Robert Lent of the University of Rio De Janeiro seems to have given us the best answer to date. Their technique involved taking whole brains and dissolving them into a suspension. The dissolving process broke down most cell structures but kept the nucleus of each cell intact.[52]

A suspension is a mixture of particles in a solvent, where the particles are large enough to settle out. However, this suspension of dissolved brain was kept uniform by intense agitation. Since each cell in the brain has exactly one nucleus, the total number of cells would be equal to the number of nuclei. The researchers drew off a sample and counted the number of nuclei. Now, knowing the density of the cells in the sample, they multiplied the density by the total volume of the dissolved brain. This yielded the total number of brain cells.

One final problem remains, not all brain cells are neurons, there are many supporting cells, called glia, in the brain. Fortunately, it is possible to distinguish between these neural and glial nuclei with a special antibody. This antibody binds only to the nuclei of neurons. Thus, it was possible to determine what percentage of total brain cells were neurons.

From this procedure, our best estimate of total neurons in the adult male human brain is 86.1 billion.[53]

Most neurons are synaptically interfaced with thousands of other neurons. This means that, despite their enormous number, between any two neurons there are, on average, only six or seven separating neurons.[54]

Long Term Potentiation

From Kandel's work we learned that the memory trace is a change in the connections between neurons. While there are undoubtedly a number of processes at work, the best understood is long term potentiation. In long term potentiation, repetitive stimulation of a neuron increases its efficiency. The increase of efficiency takes the form of an increase in the amount of neurotransmitter released. Significantly, this change in efficiency continues after the stimulation has ceased. Thus, information can be stored in configurations of neurons as different levels of synaptic efficiency.[55]

One important feature of long term potentiation is associativity. A neuron's efficiency can be changed by the combined synchronized stimulation of two other neurons. Thus, two or more neuronal inputs can become associated with each other according to some computational process. [56] This suggests that the associative structure of memory, a topic central is memory improvement, is rooted in the brains underlying biology.

In addition to the potentiation of neurons, there also two briefer process: facilitation and augmentation. In facilitation, the neuron's increase in efficiency lasts for a fraction of a second, while in augmentation it lasts for a few seconds.[57]

It does not take much imagination to see that short term memories may be stored as temporary patterns of facilitation and augmentation, while long term memories are stored as long term potentiation of neurons.

Halle Berry Neurons

Our most direct evidence for the existence of the memory trace comes from research conducted on patients with epilepsy by Rodrigo Quian Quiroga and his colleagues.[58] Normally epilepsy is controlled by medications, unfortunately, drugs do not always work, and some patients require brain surgery. Surgeons either remove the brain tissue where seizures begin, or they cut the neural pathways that spread seizure activity. Successful surgery depends on correctly locating the source of the seizure. Non-invasive techniques such as EEG are not always successful and in these cases the doctors will implant electrodes directly into the brain to find the seizure focus. The electrodes usually remain in place for several days. This intervention allowed researchers to directly monitor how the brain responds to specific stimuli. Eight volunteer, all patients with implanted electrodes as part of their treatment for epilepsy, agreed to participate in an experimental study. While lying in a bed, they were shown a series of images on a computer screen. In rapid succession the volunteers were shown pictures of buildings, animals, and famous people. Occasionally, a spike of neuron activity would occur at one of the electrodes in response to an image. For example, when one volunteer was shown a picture of actress Halle Berry, a group of neurons located in the front of the right hippocampus would show a significant increase in activity. When the volunteer was shown other images of Halle Berry, playing Catwoman, for example, the same neurons would activate. These neurons would not activate if show a generic picture of Catwoman, not played by Halle Berry. This same group of neurons, however, would activate to the printed name "Halle Berry." This was direct evidence of a localized memory trace.

Knowing something of the biological background of memory will help us answer the question posed in the next chapter, can memory be improved?

1   Gardner, M. (1988). *Hexaflexagons and other
    metamathematical diversions*. Chicago: University
    of Chicago Press.
2   Hilgard, E. R. & Bower, G. H. (1975). *Theories of
    learning* (4th edition). Englewood Cliffs, NJ:
    Prentice-Hall, Inc.
3   Abramson, C. I. (1994). *A primer of invertebrate
    learning: The behavioral perspective.* Washington,
    DC: American Psychological Association.
4   Andreassi, J. L. (1995). *Psychophysiology: Human
    behavior and physiological response.* Hillsdale, NJ:
    Lawrence Erlbaum Associates.
5   Lykken, D. T. (1995). The antisocial personalities.
    Hillsdale, NJ: Lawrence Erlbaum Associates,
    Publishers.
6   Woodruff-Pak, D. .S., Finkbiner, R. G., & Sasse, D.
    K. (1990). *Neuroreport, 1,* 45 - 48.
7   Powell, R. A., Symbaluk, D. G., & Honey, P. L.
    (2009). *Introduction to learning and behavior.* 3rd
    Ed. Belmont, CA: Warsworth.
8   Dykman, R. A., Ackerman, P. T., & Newton J. E. O.
    (1997). Posttraumatic stress disorder: A
    sensitization reaction. *Integrative Physiological
    and Behavioral Science, 32,* 9 - 18.
9   Catania, A. C. (1998). *Learning* (4th edition).
    Upper Saddle River, NJ: Prentice Hall. p. 319
10 Dudai, Y. (1989). *The neurobiology of memory:*

Concepts, findings, trends. Oxford: Oxford University Press. p. 6

11 Tolman,E. C. (1958). Behavior and psychological man. Berkeley, CA: University of California Press.

12 Thorndike, E. L. (1913). *Educational Psychology: Volume II; The original nature of man.* New York: Teachers College, Columbia University.

13 Tolman,E. C. (1958). Behavior and psychological man. Berkeley, CA: University of California Press. p. 247

[14] Donahoe, J. W. & Palmer, D. C. (1994). *Learning and complex behavior.* Boston: Allyn and Bacon.

[15] Fuster, J. M. (1999). *Memory in the cerebral cortex.* Cambridge, MA: MIT Press.

[16] Montessori, M. (1967). *The absorbent mind.* Cutchogue, NY: Buccaneer Books.

[17] Garcia, J., & Garcia Y Robertson, R. (1985). Evolution of learning mechanisms. In B. L. Hammonds (Ed.). *Psychology and Learning* (pp. 191 - 243). Washington, DC: American Psychological Association. p. 223

[18] Norman, D. A. (1969). *Memory and attention: An introduction to human information processing.* New York: John Wiley & Sons.

[19] Thompson, R. F., & Madigan, S. A. (2005). *Memory: The key to consciousness. Washington,* D.C.: Joseph Henry Press.

[20] Baxendale, S. (2010). The Flynn effect and memory

function. *Journal of Clinical and Experimental Neuropsychology, 32,* 699 - 703.

[21] Baddeley, A., Eysenck, M. W., & Anderson, M. C. (2010). *Memory.* New York: Psychology Press

[22] Schwartz, B. L. (2011). *Memory: Foundations and applications.* Los Angeles, CA: Sage Publications.

[23] Miller, G. A. (1956). The magical number seven, plus or minus two: some limits on our capacity for processing information. *Psychological review, 63*(2), 81 - 97.

[24] Schwartz, B. L. (2011). *Memory: Foundations and applications.* Los Angeles, CA: Sage Publications.

[25] Ellis, N. C., & Hennelly, R. A. (1980). A bilingual word-length effect: Implications for intelligence testing and the relative ease of mental calculations in Welsh and English. *British Journal of Psychology, 71,* 43 - 51.

[26] Hebb, D. O. (1949). *The organization of behavior: A neurophysical theory.* New York: John Wiley & Sons.

[27] Howard, R. W. (1995) Learning and memory: Major ideas, principles, issues and applications. Westport, CT: Praeger.

[28] Dudai, Y. (2002). *Memory: From A to Z.* Oxford; Oxford University Press.

Eysenck, H. J., & Eysenck, M. W. (Eds.). (1994).

Mind watching : Why we behave the way we do.
London: Smithmark Publishers.

[29] Zola-Morgan, S. & Squire, L. R. (1993). The memory
system damaged in medial temporal lobe amnesia:
Findings from humans and nonhuman primates.
In T. Ono et al. (Eds). *Brain mechanisms of
perception and memory: From neuron to behavior*
(pp. 241 – 257). New York: Oxford University Press.

[30] Shenk, D. (2003). *The forgetting: Alzheimer's:
Portrait of an epidemic.* New York: Anchor
Books

[31] Maguire, E. A., Woollett, K. & Spiers, H. J. (2006).
London taxi drivers and bus drivers: A structural
MRI and neuropsychological analysis.
Hippocampus, 16: 1091 - 1101.

[32] Dudai, Y. (2002). *Memory: From A to Z.* Oxford;
Oxford University Press.

[33] Hebb, D. O. (1949). *The organization of behavior: A
neurophysical theory.* New York: John Wiley &
Sons.

[34] Kandel, E. R. & Hawkins, R. D. (1993). The
biological basis of learning and individuality. In
Mind and brain: Readings from Scientific
American magazine. (Pp. 40 - 53).

[35] Kandel, E. R. & Hawkins, R. D. (1993). The
biological basis of learning and individuality. In
Mind and brain: Readings from Scientific

American magazine. (Pp. 40 - 53).

[36] Sharp, P. E. (1993). The role of the hippocampus in learning and memory. In T. Ono et al. (Eds). *Brain mechanisms of perception and memory: From neuron to behavior* (pp. 370 – 393). New York: Oxford University Press.

[37] Dudai, Y. (2002). *Memory: From A to Z*. Oxford; Oxford University Press.

[38] Shenk, D. (2003). *The forgetting: Alzheimer's: Portrait of an epidemic*. New York: Anchor Books.

[39] McConnell, J. V. (Ed.), (1967). *A manual of psychological experimentation on planarians*. Ann Arbor, MI: The Worm Runner's Digest.

[40] Rilling, M. (1996). The mystery of the vanished citation: James McConnell's forgotten quest for planarian learning, a biochemical engram, and celebrity. *American Psychologist, 51,* 589 - 598.

[41] Collins, H, & Pinch, T. (1993). *The Golem: What everyone should know about science*. Cambridge, UK: Cambridge University Press.

[42] Rilling, M. (1996). The mystery of the vanished citation: James McConnell's forgotten quest for planarian learning, a biochemical engram, and celebrity. *American Psychologist, 51,* 589 - 598.

[43] Hobson, J. A. (1988). *The dreaming brain*. New York: Basic Books.

[44] Gerard, R. W. (1953/1971). What is memory. In R. F.

Thompson (Ed.) *Physiological psychology.* (pp. 372 -377). San Francisco: W. H. Freeman and Company.

[45] Gerard, R. W. (1953/1971). What is memory. In R. F. Thompson (Ed.) *Physiological psychology.* (pp. 372 -377). San Francisco: W. H. Freeman and Company. (p. 375).

[46] Rosenzweig, M. R., & Bennett, E. L. (1996). Psychobiology of plasticity: The effects of training and experience on brain and behavior. *Behavioural Brain Research, 78,* 57 - 65.

[47] Rosenzweig, M. R., & Bennett, E. L. (1996). Psychobiology of plasticity: The effects of training and experience on brain and behavior. *Behavioural Brain Research, 78,* 57 - 65.

[48] Squire, L. R. (1987). *Memory and brain.* New York: Oxford University Press.

[49] Buchsbaum, R. et al. (1987). *Animals without backbones.* Chicago: University of Chicago Press.

[50] Thompson, R. F., & Madigan, S. A. (2005). *Memory: The key to consciousness. Washington,* D.C.: Joseph Henry Press.

[51] Kandel, E. R., Schwartz, J. H., & Jessell, T. M. (Eds.). (2000). *Principles of neural science* (Vol. 4). New York: McGraw-Hill.

[52] Herculano-Houzel, S., & Lent, R. (2005). Isotropic

fractionator: A simple, rapid method for the quantification of total cell and neuronal numbers in the brain. *The Journal of Neuroscience, 25,* 2518 - 2521.

[53] Azevedo, F. A. C., et al., (2009). Equal numbers of neuronal and nonneuronal cells make the human brain an isometrically scaled-up primate brain. *The Journal of Comparative Neurology, 513,* 532 - 541.

[54] Baars, B. J. (1988) *A cognitive theory of consciousness.* Cambridge, UK: Cambridge University Press.

[55] Dudai, Y. (1989). *The neurobiology of memory: Concepts, findings, trends.* Oxford: Oxford University Press.

[56] Holscher, C. (2001). Introduction; Long-term potentiation\as a model for memory mechanism: The story so far. In C. Holscher (Ed.). *Neuronal mechanisms of memory formation: Concepts of long-term potentiation and beyond.* (pp. 1 -34). Cambridge, UK: Cambridge University Press.

[57] Dudai, Y. (1989). *The neurobiology of memory: Concepts, findings, trends.* Oxford: Oxford University Press.

[58] Quiroga, R. Q. et al. (2005). Invariant visual representation by single neurons in the human brain. *Nature, 435,* 1102 - 1107.

Chapter 4

Is Memory Improvement Possible?

We usually have a very positive view of ourselves. When asked to compare themselves with others on such desirable traits as intelligence, generosity, or leadership skills, most people rate themselves as above average, a mathematical impossibility.[1] Athletic performance and memory are the exceptions. Most of us know we are not star athletes, and most of us believe that we have poor memories.[2] Perhaps this anomaly is caused by the nature of the feedback the world provides. Our friends are loath to set us straight about our generosity. They may feel it impolite to relate their true feelings about our intelligence. Athletic and memory feedback, however, come to us more directly. If we start the race thinking we can finish first, our expectation will soon be confirmed or disproved. Similarly, a memory failure can be direct, immediate, often visible to all, and, sometimes, deeply embarrassing.[3] Moreover, as we get older, memory failure stirs up deep fears of mental frailty and impending senility.

I have good news. It is unlikely that you have a poor memory, rather you have a memory that can be improved. In this chapter, I will try to demonstrate the possibility of memory improvement. First, I must spend some time addressing a fundamental question, is memory skill a matter of nature or nurture? Is someone just born with a good memory or is it the result of practice and training?

There clearly are people who learn faster than others and people with extraordinary powers of recall. Examples of powerful memories include, maestro Arturo Toscanini, who conducted complex symphonies without written scores and Kim Peek, a savant who could remember everything he read and was the model for the title character in the film *Rain Man*.[4]

Because he was portrayed be Dustin Hoffman in the film *Rain Man*, many people are familiar with Kim Peek's remarkable abilities. For example, Peek, who died in 2009, could remember the verbatim contents of an entire book years after a single reading. In Peek's case his extraordinary memory must have been related to factors present at birth, particularly his unique brain structure. The corpus callosum, a fibrous band of neurons that normally connect the two brain hemispheres, was missing altogether, and he had a malformed cerebellum.[5] He also had significant social and motor deficits and did not walk until he was four years old. It is believed Peek had a genetic disorder called FG syndrome, caused by a defect on the X chromosome.[6]

Other examples of powerful memories are hyperpolyglots, individuals who speak many languages. Linguist Michael Erard defines a hyperpolyglot as someone who can speak (or read, write, or translate) at least eleven languages although other use a less strict criterion of six languages. For example, Erard describes Johan Vanderwalle, head of the Turkish-language department at Ghent University. In a public test of his skill, Vanderwalle was certified competent in 19 languages. There is controversy of the origin of such impressive ability. Do hyper-polyglots have a greater natural ability for language learning? Or are they simply more motivated to spend the requisite amount of time studying?[7]

On the other hand, we know that there are people who suffer from pathological memory problems such as amnesia or dementia. Patients with late stage Alzheimer's dementia forget their own identity and loss their language skills.[8] So, clearly, some people do have substantially impaired memory ability.

Technique or Talent?

For most of us, it is safe to assume that we have ordinary memory ability. Ordinary, however, is nothing to scoff at. The storage capacity of even a normal memory is enormous. For example, most of us know thousands of words that we can summon rapidly. More to the point, there is good evidence that we can substantially improve our memory performance through technique and practice.

Take the case of journalist Joshua Foer, who became America's memory champion after only a year of practice. Memory competitions have proliferated, and America crowns its memory champion every March. Foer had covered the U.S. Memory Championship as a reporter for Slate.com. He was struck by the insistence of most competitors that they did not have particularly good memories but, instead, employed well practiced mnemonic techniques. In his fascinating book, *Moonwalking with Einstein,* he details his near obsessive attempt to master memory techniques and compete for the memory championship. Among other feats Foer learned to memorize the order of a shuffled deck of cards in a minute and 40 seconds.[9]

The ancients are often credited with having tremendous powers of memory. Themistocles, a Greek general and politician, who lived around 500 B.C.E., remembered the names of 20,000 Athenians.[10] While it is impossible to know for certain, this amazing claim is plausible. Themistocles may have employed a mnemonic system. We can infer this from two lines of evidence. First, such systems were popular in antiquity. Second, we know that the contemporary memory performer Harry Lorayne has committed millions of names and faces to memory over the course of a 40 year career using memory techniques.[11]

Hideaki Tomoyori set a world record for memorizing digits of the irrational number pi in 1987. He recited 40,000 digits in 786 minutes. One might think Tomoyori was born with a powerful memory, but tests revealed he did not seem to have superior cognitive abilities. Rather his amazing feat was accomplished through mnemonic techniques and extensive practice. While memorizing digits of pi is, undoubtedly, an arcane pursuit, we will see that the same mnemonic techniques can be applied to help us with many practical memory problems.[12]

A study, by researcher Eleanor Maguire and her colleagues, compared ten individuals with superior memories, included in the sample were eight high level performers at the World Memory Championship, with ten matched controls. The two groups had similar levels of cognitive ability. Magnetic resonance imaging of their brains revealed no structural brain differences between the superior memorizers and controls. The authors concluded that the main difference between the two groups was that the superior memorizers used mnemonic techniques.[13]

On the other hand, John Wilding and Elisabeth Valentine, psychologists at the Royal Holloway, University of London, argued for the existence of two different classes of superior memory performance: naturals, those who seem to have a naturally strong memory, and strategists, those who employ learn-ed memory strategies.[14]

This has been a controversial claim. There are certainly examples of families of who shared strong powers of memory. The historian Thomas Babington Macaulay, said to be able to memorize an entire book on a single reading, had both a father and grandfather with similar abilities.[15] However, such cases do not prove genetic ability. Families pass down much more than genes, they also pass down traditions, values, and training. We do not know if Mozart's talents came from the genes he inherited from his musical family or from the intensive musical education they provided. Some researchers have gone so far to assert that there are no naturals and all superior performance rests on the use of strategies. In *Moonwalking with Einstein* Jonathan Foer reported evidence that Daniel Tammet, who has been said to possess savant-like memory ability, may have actually used memory strategies available to anyone.[16]

Tammet's feats include learning to speak Icelandic

in one week and memorizing 22,514 digits of pi. Several respected scientists have vouched for his abilities.[17] However, memory champions like Dominic O'Brien have observed Tammet and believe that he uses standard mnemonic techniques.[18] Whatever the status of this case, there certainly have been individuals who memory performance seems to be the result of natural talent.

There is the famous case of Solomon Sherashevsky discovered by the Russian neuropsychologist A. R. Luria. Sherashevsky grew up in a small Russian Jewish community. The earliest indication that there was something different about Sherashevsky was his experience of synesthesia, a neurological condition where a person experiences automatic associations between sensory modalities. For, example, someone with synesthesia might experience strong color associations with certain sounds. Sherashevsky told Luria that, as a child of two or three, he experienced the words of a Hebrew prayer as "puffs of steam or splashes."[19] Even as an adult certain sounds would produce those same images.

At an early age, Sherashevsky showed musical aptitude, but an ear disease impaired his hearing and he had to give up his musical ambitions. He tried to work as a newspaper reporter. His editor noticed that Sherashevsky never took notes when he gave out the days assignments. Since the assignments were often complicated, the editor chastised Sherashevsky for inattention. Sherashevsky startled his editor by repeating back the day's assignment verbatim. The editor sent Sherashevsky to Luria's laboratory to have his memory tested.

One of the first things to strike Luria was that Sherashevsky "wasn't aware of any peculiarities in himself and couldn't conceive of the idea that his memory differed in some way from other people's."[20]

Luria started testing Sherashevsky's memory. His first instinct was to find the limits of Sherashevsky ability. Luria read of lists of numbers and words. But, no matter how long the list Sherashevsky succeeded in repeating it back. This was startling because the classic research on memory by Ebbinghaus had found that the ability to recall a list declines as the list grows longer.[21] Luria came to the conclusion that Sherashevsky's memory "had no distinct limits."[22] According to Luria "all he required was that there be a three-to-four second pause between each element in the series, and he had no difficulty responding whatever I gave him."[23] It made no difference if lists were of words, numbers, sounds, or nonsense syllables, Sherashevsky remembered them all. Indeed, they seemed to become a part of his long term memory; Luria found that Sherashevsky could recall the lists when retested fifteen years later.

And yet, while Sherashevsky might seem the perfect case of a naturally superior memory, Luria discovered that he employed a technique very much like the method of loci found in most memory improvement books. In the method of loci, one uses a series of well remembered locations usually arranged in a journey, as hooks to attach new information. According to Luria, when Sherashevsky read through a long series of words, each word would require a graphic image. And since the series was fairly long, he had to find some way of distinguishing these images of his in a mental row of sequences. Most often (and this habit persisted throughout his life), he would 'distribute' them along some roadway or street he visualized in his mind.[24]

Sherashevsky appears to have self discovered the method of loci. How are we to interpret the fact that Sherashevsky used a memory technique? Was his skill the result of training, natural ability, or some combination of both?

One way we might answer this question is to see if ordinary people could be trained to duplicate impressive feats of memory. For example, Sherashevsky was able to memorize a large matrix of 50 numbers arranged in 12 rows of four digits and one row of two digits. This seems a task beyond the reach of most people.

Yet, Kenneth Higbee, a psychology professor at Brigham Young University, was able to train ordinary college students to duplicate Sherashevsky's feat using a mnemonic system called the phonetic alphabet to learn the same matrix. We will learn a version of the phonetic alphabet in Chapter 7. The students in Higbee's study were able to learn the matrix in three minutes, the same time it took Sherashevsky.[25]

It remains possible, however, that Sherashevsky had some power beyond that of technique. For one thing, while Higbee's students were able to duplicate Sherashevsky's in immediately recalling the list, his complete performance was still more impressive. Sherashevsky was also able to recall the list in reverse order and the numbers in individual columns. Indeed, he could recite the numbers in zig zag diagonals through the chart.[26]

It certainly seems likely that with additional practice the students would have obtained Sherashevsky like levels of performance. However, one wonders if they would, as Sherashevsky could, recall the list years later.

Our best explanation for Sherashevsky may be some combination of innate skill and technique. It seems possible that Sherashevsky's synesthesia gave him superior powers of mental imaging that he harnessed to an age old memory technique. Research has shown that synesthesia is a real phenomenon. For example, some people with synesthesia see numbers as having specific colors. The physician and neuroscientist V.R. Ramachandran recruited two people who saw the number five as green and the number two as red. He created a computerized test that presented a group of twos arranged in a geometric shape embedded in a random display of fives. The two people with synesthesia were able immediately to discern the shape formed by the twos. People without synesthesia took as long as 20 seconds to find the shape.[27]

Synesthesia is involuntary, develops early in life, and seems to be genetic in origin. [28] Thus, Sherashevsky's skill may have involved both natural ability and technique.[29] Later Sherashevsky became a professional memory performer and learned to use standard mnemonic techniques.

One peculiarity of Sherashevsky was that, while his synesthesia gave him great powers of visualization, he had difficulty noticing the meaningful structure of the material he memorized. Luria once gave him a long series of numbers to memorize.

1234
2345
3456
4567
etc.

Luria reports that it took Sherashevsky an "intense effort" and that he was "unaware that the numbers in the series progressed in a simple logical order."[30]

Mr. Memory

A remarkable example of exceptional memory was the English music hall sensation, W. J. M. Bottle, who performed under the stage name Datas. He could recall thousands of obscure facts. Bottle, who was the inspiration for the Mr. Memory character in Alfred Hitchcock's film *The 39 steps*, could answer trivia questions shouted from the audience, The ages and birthdays of celebrities, the results of sporting matches, obscure facts of geography; his range of knowledge was astounding.[31] Bottle wrote a memoir where he disclaimed any early knowledge of special memory powers. In the same book he tells of his accidental discovery of his powerful memory when he overheard two men trying to remember the date of the verdict in the Tichborne trial, a notorious Victorian scandal.[32]

Heir to a great fortune Roger Tichborne had been lost at sea and pronounced dead. An Australian butcher named Arthur Orton, who bore only a slight resemblance to the missing man, came forward and claimed to be Tichborne. Orton's claim was accepted by Tichborne's mother, but after her death Orton tried to claim the inheritance. His bid failed and he was eventually convicted of perjury.

Bottle provided the date of Orton's conviction, February 28, 1874. When one of the men expressed surprise that Bottle would know a date of an event that occurred before his birth, Bottle proceeded to provide all the important details of the Tichborne case

In his memoir, Bottle tells us "finding how surprised they were at my stock of knowledge, I felt encouraged, and continued with a number of dates of events in English history, and the names of Derby and Oaks' winners, in rapid succession." [33] Bottle's performance was overheard by a theatrical promoter who invited him to appear on the Standard Music Hall that very night, Still dressed in his dirty work clothes, Bottle was an instant success and soon quit his job as a manual laborer at a gas works for a life in show business.

Reading Bottle's autobiography one finds evidence that Bottle may have had Asperger's syndrome, an autism spectrum disorder characterized by social awkwardness and obsessive interest in facts and details. Many children with Asperger's syndrome are hyperlexic, teaching themselves to read at an early age.[34] Bottle had scant schooling and taught himself to read. As a child he showed obsessive interest in obscure facts, "from memorizing shop-keepers' names I got to cabbies' and policeman's number."[35] Like most children with Asperger's syndrome he took little interest in his peers. "I was not the same as most other children, in that I took no part in their games, having no desire to."[36]

Bottle had great powers of visualization and he may have had synesthesia. However, in his memoir he specifically rejected any claim to have an extraordinary memory. Yet, he also claimed not to employ mnemonic techniques.

So where does this leave us? It seems clear that Kim Peek was biologically endowed with a superior memory. The cases of Sherashevsky and Bottle is less clear. No scientific evaluation of Bottle was ever published and we know that Sherashevsky, did at least sometimes, employee mnemonic techniques. Whatever the status of these cases we do have evidence that the some people have naturally superior memory talents while others have ordinary memory trained to perform at very high levels. We call this the natural — strategist distinction. In 1994, researchers John Wilding and Elizabeth Valentine ran extensive tests on a group of superior memorizers. Some of the tests, such as memorizing six telephone number each six digit longs and each associated with a person's name, lent themselves to the use of mnemonic techniques. Other tests, for example, recognizing 14 previously seen pictures of snowflakes out of a field of 70 snowflakes never seen before, did not, in any obvious way, lend themselves to a strategy.

The participants included some individuals who were identified as memory strategists, for example, "subject C began to learn memory techniques and practice intensively about four years before we met him and uses mainly the method of loci." Other participants seemed to posses natural memory abilities; "subject D was one of the rare female subjects in this area of study, working as journalist. She said that she found it easy to memorize material at school and was good at languages, including mastering accent, but not at spatial relations, her sense of direction being poor. She reported that several near relatives had exceptionally good memories." [37] Wilding and Valentine classified individuals as natural memorizers if they reported having a good memory from early childhood and had at least one relative with an exceptional memory.

On average the natural memorizers outperformed the strategic memorizers on tasks like identifying snowflakes, while the memory strategists outperformed the memory naturals on tasks that lent themselves to a mnemonic method, such as memorizing lists of phone numbers. We can draw two conclusions from this research. First, there are people who do have natural memory abilities. Second, that people with ordinary memory, using mnemonic techniques, can sometimes outperform people with superior natural ability.

Imitating Bubbles P.

Psychologist K. Anders Ericsson is the leading authority on how people develop expertise. He is also skeptical about claims of naturally superior memory. Ericsson wanted to see if it was possible to train individuals with normal memories to duplicate the feats of savants and memory performers.

One remarkable feat is the ability of some to hold large amounts of information in short term memory.

Most of us can hold only about 7 digits in short term memory. Yet there have been some impressive examples of individuals who have far exceeded this limit. In one case, a Philadelphia gambler, known in the research literature as Bubbles P., was able to hold 15 to 20 digits in his short term memory.[38] This was the type of performance Ericsson wanted to duplicate.

In Ericsson's experiment, an average college student practiced memorizing strings of digits for one hour a day several days a week. After 230 hours of practice the student's digit span ability rose to 80 digits. The student accomplished this task by developing a mnemonic strategy that transformed groups of digits into chunks. We can think of a chunk as a unit of information. When we say that on average we can hold only 7 digits in our short term memory, we would be more correct to say that we hold 7 chunks, each chunk in turn holding only one digit of information. The distinction is important because a chunk can be made to bear more information than a single digit. For example, if we remember 3 and 6 as single digits each digit is a separate chunk. If, however, we combine them into the single number 36, it becomes as single chunk.

The student who participated in Ericsson's study was a competitive runner and he found that he could think of many 3 or 4 digit sequences as running times. Thus, for most of us the digit sequence 3492 would be held in our short term memory as four chunks, he was able to see the sequence as a 3 minutes and 49.2 time in a mile race. For him 3492 became a single chunk. Since some number strings are easily converted to running times and some are not Ericsson was able to study the effectiveness of this chunking strategy. When the student was presented with only numbers that could be interpreted as running times he could retain, on average 19.5 digits. When given digit sequences that could not be translated into running times his performance fell to near his beginning level. Over time, he invented additional chunking strategies that boosted his performance to 80 digits.[39]

One does not have to share Ericsson's skepticism about natural memory to realize the significance of this research. This supports the central doctrine of memory improvement: high levels of memory performance are possible with training. Many memory strategists claim to have normal or even below normal natural memories. Dominic O'Brien was diagnosed with dyslexia and did poorly in school, yet became the world memory champion.[40] Tony Buzan writes that, as a student, he "only occasionally performed well" on exams.[41] After learning mnemonic strategies, he graduated from the University of British Columbia with honors in psychology, English, mathematics, and general science. Harry Lorayne, who could memorize thousands of names, writes that his memory "was no better or worse than most people's."[42]

The Capacity of Long Term Memory

In his accounts of his friendship with the great detective Sherlock Holmes, Watson is surprised to learn of Holmes' lack of basic knowledge:

His ignorance was as remarkable as his knowledge. Of contemporary literature, philosophy and politics he appeared to know next to nothing. Upon my quoting Thomas Carlyle, he inquired in the naivest way who he might be and what he had done. My surprise reached a climax, however, when I found incidentally that he was ignorant of the Copernican Theory and of the composition of the Solar System. That any civilized human being in this nineteenth century should not be aware that the earth traveled round the sun appeared to be to me such an extraordinary fact that I could hardly realize it.

"You appear to be astonished," he said, smiling at my expression of surprise. "Now that I do know it I shall do my best to forget it."

"To forget it!"

"You see," he explained, "I consider that a man's brain originally is like a little empty attic, and you have to stock it with such furniture as you choose. A fool takes in all the lumber of every sort that he comes across, so that the knowledge which might be useful to him gets crowded out, or at best is jumbled up with a lot of other things so that he has a difficulty in laying his hands upon it. Now the skillful workman is very careful indeed as to what he takes into his brain-attic. He will have nothing but the tools which may help him in doing his work, but of these he has a large assortment, and all in the most perfect order. It is a mistake to think that that little room has elastic walls and can distend to any extent. Depend upon it there comes a time when for every addition of knowledge you forget something that you knew before."[43]

Holmes was not alone in this belief. There is an apocryphal story about a professor of ichthyology who complained every time he had to learn a student's name he forgot the name of a fish.[44] We could call this the attic theory of memory, the belief that our long term memory has some approachable limit. According to this idea, every fact is learned at the expense of some other fact.

There was a running gag on the popular old time radio comedy *Fibber McGee and Molly*, when an overstuffed closet would be opened and pour out its contents. Our memory is not an attic, nor is it Fibber McGee's closet. It is neither disorganized or overstuffed.

Holmes and the ichthyologist were mistaken. The already impressive powers of Holmes would have been enhanced with greater knowledge. Fish and students could rest comfortably together in the ichthyologist's long term memory.

We know this from several lines of evidence. As I have already mentioned studies of memory demonstrate that increased knowledge improves memory. A fact that directly refutes the attic theory.

In addition, the vast connective architecture of the brain, with its billions of connections, suggests a gigantic storage capacity. We describe the storage capacity of computers in terms of bits. A bit is the smallest possible unit of information, essentially the answer to a true or false question, represented as a zero (for no) or a one (for yes).[45]

How many bits could the human brain store? We could estimate this by the total number of connections between neurons. Each connection counting as one bit. Using this procedure, scientists have estimated that the human brain can store 10^{8432} bits of information.[46] That is one followed by 8,432 zeros. If this number is correct, it means that a single human brain has more storage capacity than all the digital computers in the world. However, this estimation rests on the assumption that the brain contains 100 billion neurons, and recent research has suggested that number is closer to 86.1 billion.[47] Even with a smaller value, the number of connections in our brain is unfathomably large.

A famous experiment conducted by Roger Shepard at Bell Labs gives us some sense of the memory's huge capacity. Volunteers from the lab's technical and clerical staff were shown 612 slides, mostly of single objects, the volunteer could advance the slides at a self-paced rate. Several days after working through all the slides, the participants were shown side by side pairs of images. In each pair, one image was drawn from those already seen, and one image was a new. They had to indicate which picture they had already seen. The participants average 87% correct answers.[48]

Finally we have examples of people of ordinary intelligence who are fluent in several languages. People who live in parts of the world where several languages are spoken, often learn more than one language. A multilingual person must have enormous vocabularies stored in long term memory.

Attention: Memory's Prerequisite

In his book on memory Ian Hunter gives a striking example of memory failure. A teacher read a short poem several times and asked his students to try to commit it to memory. After many readings, his pupils succeeded in learning the verses. The teacher, however, was dismayed when he realized that he had not learned the poem![49]

Attention is a prerequisite for memory and many events that we interpret as memory failures are actually failures of attention. At any instant, a vast flood of information streams into our central nervous system. Photons strike the retinas of our eyes, sound waves cause our eardrums to vibrate, tactile neurons are stimulated by the feel of clothes on our body, all of this sensory information passes into our brain. This is the preattentive or sensory memory I have already described. Yet we are only aware of a small amount of this information.

We must focus or be overwhelmed. We call this focusing attention. Attention is a limited resource, it can be strained to the breaking point. This is the reason we must turn down the car radio when we seek an unknown address. We have all had the experience of talking to a perfectly nice person at a party, only to discover that some other conversation is much more interesting than the one we are stuck in. We have to struggle to maintain focus and continue attending to the less interesting words of our conversational partner.

The things that we attend to are the things of which we are aware. Awareness is the front end of the memory system, and if we do not pay attention to information, it will never enter the memory system. Information that is not attended to, or that is processed in a habitual or automatic fashion without awareness, will not be remembered.[50]

Why did we forget where we parked the car? Because when we arrived at the mall we were preoccupied (the kids were screaming, we were in a hurry, and so on) and did not pay attention to where we parked. If we had made a point of noting where we parked on arrival ("to the left of the Trader Joe's, just near the food court entrance") there would be a much greater probability of finding the car.

Driving and parking a car are examples of an automatic, habitual processes. Over our lifetime, we learn to make many of our actions automatic, freeing up our awareness to attend to other matters. This is a very useful division of labor, but it means that we don't attend to things we do automatically and are less likely to remember them. Losing small objects, like keys, wallets, and cell phones, falls into this category. We are used to handling these things habitually without attention. Thus, we experience a high degree of forgetting of things related to routine tasks. We are so used to shutting the garage door that we do it without attention. Thus, it is not surprising that we may not recall if we actually did shut it.

There are two ways to deal with this type of forgetting. One is to engineer our habits. For example, we could designate a special place for our keys, say a hook in the bedroom, where we always hang them up at the end of the day.

The other approach is to disrupt our habitual processing, cueing ourselves to pay attention at a critical moment. We can use this approach to help us remember names.

Lack of attention helps to explain why we have

such difficulty remembering names. It is true that names are particularly difficult to remember. We tend to be good at recognizing faces ("I know that I know that person"), but bad at associating the correct name with the face. Like all primates we devote a large part of our cortex to processing visual information, we are visually dominant. But matching a name with a face, that is matching visual with auditory information, requires the complex coordination across a number of brain areas. However difficult the task of remembering names, it is rendered impossible if we never learned the name in the first place. You know the drill. You are introduced to someone, often in a stressful situation such as the first day of work. You are distracted and do not catch the name. The next time you meet you are too embarrassed to admit you did not learn the name, a problem that compounds with time. One could spend an entire career not knowing the name of a coworker. Harry Lorayne joked that we can think of such cases of forgetting as "not getting."[51]

The alternative is to make sure you learn the name on the first day by disrupting the normal pattern of inattention. Pay attention to the name. Make a point of repeating the name when first introduced. If appropriate ask about pronunciation and spelling. Use the person's name in the conversation and when you say goodbye. While not a guarantee, these simple procedures will increase the probability of remembering.[52]

In a highly influential paper (Google Scholar shows that it has been cited 6,222 times as of this writing) Fergus Craik and Robert Lockhart argued that attention's link to memory can be understood in terms of different levels of processing. There is a type I processing that attends only to the superficial characteristics of an object or event, such as its physical and sensory characteristics. If we process information only at this superficial level and it is less likely to enter longterm memory.

Type II processing is said to have a greater depth because it pays attention to the meaning of new information. In Type II processing we try to make connections between the new information and information already in our long term memory. This is sometimes called elaborative processing and is associated with superior remembering. A student who is focused on the teacher's accent is engaged in type I processing, and is unlikely to remember much from the lecture. Attending to meaning, type II processing, is creating long term memories.[53]

If attention is so important to memory then training our attention must be an important component of any effort to improve memory.[54] Efforts to train attention can be traced back to ancient times. Dharana, the practice of "binding the mind to one place, object or idea,"[55] was designated as fifth of yoga's eight limbs in the Yoga Sutras. Dharana is sometimes translated as concentration. The yogis developed a number of techniques for strengthening attention through concentration and meditation.

Modern science gives some support to these techniques. Meditation and mindfulness training have been shown to improve attention.[56] Thus, it makes sense to include meditation as part of your memory improvement strategy. Many excellent books and meditation programs are available. I recommend *The Miracle of Mindfulness* by Buddhist monk Thich Nhat Hanh as a good introduction.[57]

Memory improvement books have always recognized the importance of improving attention and often propose exercises. Harry Lorayne recommends that when you see someone on a bus or in a waiting room, "close your eyes and try to mentally describe every detail of this person's face. ...(then) check yourself. You'll find your observation getting finer each time your try it."[58]

One book recommends glancing at random three to four letter words on signs or in the newspaper, closing your eyes and trying to visualize the word spelled backwards. As your ability improves, you are advised to try progressively longer words. Unfortunately, most of these techniques have not been rigorously tested and, at this point, we must remain agnostic about their effectiveness.[59]

[1] Dunning, D., Heath, C., & Suls, J. M. (2004) Flawed self-assessment: Implications for health education, and the workplace. *Psychological Science in the Public Interest, 5,* 71 – 106.

[2] Eysenck, H. J., & Eysenck, M. W. (Eds.). (1994). *Mind watching : Why we behave the way we do.* London: Smithmark Publishers. Hunter, I. M. L, (1974).

Memory. Middlesex: England. Pelican Books.

[3] Dunning, D., Heath, C., & Suls, J. M. (2004) Flawed self-assessment: Implications for health education, and the workplace. *Psychological Science in the Public Interest, 5,* 71 – 106.

[4] Weinland, J. D. (1957). *How to improve your memory.* New York: Barnes and Noble, Inc.

[5] Treffert, D. A. & Christensen, D.D.(2005). Inside the Mind of a Savant. *Scientific American,* December, 109 - 113.

[6] Opitz, J. M., Smith, J. F., & Santoro, L. (2008). The FG Syndromes. *Advances in Pediatrics, 55,* 123–170.

[7] Erard, M. (2012). *Babel no more: The search for the world's most extraordinary language learners.* New York: Free Press.

[8] Schwartz, B. L. (2011). *Memory: Foundations and applications.* Los Angeles, CA: Sage Publications.

[9] Foer, J., (2011). *Moonwalking with Einstein, The art and science of remembering everything.* New York: The Penguin Press.

[10] Buzan, T. & Keene, R. (2005). *Buzan's book of mental world records.* Hassocks, West Sussex, UK: D & B Publishing.

[11] Lorayne, H. (1975). *Remembering people: The key to success.* New York: Warner Books.

[12] Takahashi, M., Shimizu, H., Saito, S., & Tomoyori, H. (2006). One percent ability and ninety-nine

percent perspiration: A study of a Japanese memorist. *Journal of Experimental Psychology: Learning, Memory, and Cognition, 32,* 1195-1200.

[13] Maguire, E. A., Valentine, E. R., Wilding, J. M. & Kapur, N. (2003). Routes to remembering: The brains behind superior memory. *Nature Neuroscience, 6,* 90 - 95.

[14] Wilding, J., & Valentine, E. (1997). *Superior Memory.* East Sussex, UK; Psychology Press.

[15] Barlow, F. (1952). *Mental prodigies: An enquiry into the faculties of arithmetical, chess and musical prodigies, famous memorizers, precocious children, and the like, with numerous examples of "lighting" calculators and mental magic.* New York: Philosophical Library.

[16] Foer, J., (2011). *Moonwalking with Einstein, The art and science of remembering everything.* New York: The Penguin Press.

[17] Tammet, D. (2008) *Born on a blue day: Inside the extraordinary mind of an autistic savant.* New York: Free Press.

[18] Foer, J., (2011). *Moonwalking with Einstein, The art and science of remembering everything.* New York: The Penguin Press.

[19] Luria, A. R. (1968). The mind of a mnemonist: A little book about a vast memory. Cambridge, MA: Harvard University Press. (p. 22)

[20] Luria, A. R. (1968). The mind of a mnemonist: A

little book about a vast memory. Cambridge, MA: Harvard University Press. (p. 9).

[21] Ebbinghaus, H. (1913/1964). *Memory: A contribution to experimental psychology.* (Trans. H. A. Ruger & C. E. Bussenius). New York: Dover Publications.

[22] Luria, A. R. (1968). The mind of a mnemonist: A little book about a vast memory. Cambridge, MA: Harvard University Press. (p. 11).

[23] Luria, A. R. (1968). The mind of a mnemonist: A little book about a vast memory. Cambridge, MA: Harvard University Press. (p. 11).

[24] Luria, A. R. (1968). The mind of a mnemonist: A little book about a vast memory. Cambridge, MA: Harvard University Press. (p. 32).

[25] Higbee, K. L. (1997). Novices, apprentices, and mnemonists: Acquiring expertise with the phonetic mnemonic. *Applied Cognitive Psychology, 11,* 147 - 161.

[26] Luria, A. R. (1968). The mind of a mnemonist: A little book about a vast memory. Cambridge, MA: Harvard University Press.

[27] Ramachandran, V. S. (2004). *A brief tour of human consciousness; From impostor poodles to purple numbers.* New York: Pi Press.

[28] Yaro, C. & Ward, J. (2007). Searching for Shereshevskii: What is superior about the memory

of synaesthetes. *The Quarterly Journal of Experimental Psychology, 60,* 681 - 695.

[29] Foer, J., (2011). *Moonwalking with Einstein, The art and science of remembering everything.* New York: The Penguin Press.

[30] Luria, A. R. (1968). The mind of a mnemonist: A little book about a vast memory. Cambridge, MA: Harvard University Press. (p. 59).

[31] Jay, R. (1986). *Learned pigs and fireproof women.* New York: Farrar, Straus & Giroux.

[32] Datas, (1904). *Memory: A simple system of memory training.* London: Gale & Polden.

[33] Datas, (1904). *Memory: A simple system of memory training.* London: Gale & Polden. (p. 7).

[34] Frith, U. (1989). *Autism: Explaining the enigma.* Oxford, UK: Blackwell.

[35] Datas, (1904). *Memory: A simple system of memory training.* London: Gale & Polden. (p. 15).

[36] Datas, (1904). *Memory: A simple system of memory training.* London: Gale & Polden. (p. 14).

[37] Wilding, J., & Valentine, E. (1997). *Superior Memory.* East Sussex, UK; Psychology Press. (p. 232).

[38] Ceci, S., Desimone, M., & Johnson, S. (1992). Memory in context: A case study of "Bubbles P.," a gifted but uneven memorizer. In D.J. Herrmann, H. Weingartner, A. Searleman, & C. McEvoy (Eds.). *Memory improvement: Implications for memory theory.* (pp. 169 - 186). New York: Springer-Verlag.

[39] Ericsson, K. A., & Chase, W. G., (1982). Exceptional memory. *American Scientist, 70,* 607 – 615.

[40] O'Brien, D. (2000). *Learn to remember: Practical techniques and exercises to improve your memory.* San Francisco; Chronicle Books.

[41] Buzan, T. (1991). *Use your perfect memory.* New York: Plume. (p. 7).

[42] Lorayne, H. & Lucas, J. (1974). *The memory book.* New York: Ballantine Books. (p. xiv).

[43] Doyle, A. C. (1904). A Study in Scarlet, and, the Sign of the Four. New York: Harpers & Brothers. (p. 15 -16).

[44] Wickelgren, W. A. (1977). *Learning and memory.* Englewood Cliffs, NJ: Prentice-Hall Inc.

[45] Bialynicka-Birula, I, & Bialynicka-Birula, I (2004). *Modeling reality: How computers mirror life.* Oxford: Oxford University Press.

[46] Wang, Y., Liu, D., & Wang, Y. (2003). Discovering the capacity of human memory. *Brain and Mind, 4,* 189 - 198.

[47] Azevedo, F. A. C., et al., (2009). Equal numbers of neuronal and nonneuronal cells make the human brain an isometrically scaled-up primate brain. *The Journal of Comparative Neurology, 513,* 532 - 541.

[48] Shepard, R. N. (1967). Recognition memory for words, sentences, and pictures. *Journal of verbal Learning and verbal Behavior, 6*(1), 156-163.

[49] Hunter, I. M. L, (1974). *Memory*. Middlesex: England. Pelican Books.

[50] Plude, D. (1992). Attention and memory improvement. In D.J. Herrmann, H. Weingartner, A. Searleman, & C. McEvoy (Eds.). *Memory improvement: Implications for memory theory.* (pp. 150 - 168). New York: Springer-Verlag.

[51] Lorayne, H. (1975). *Remembering people: The key to success.* New York: Warner Books. (p. 20).

[52] Lorayne, H. (1975). *Remembering people: The key to success.* New York: Warner Books.

[53] Craik, F. I. M., & Lockhart, R. S. (1972). Levels of processing: A framework for memory research. *Journal of Verbal Learning and Verbal Behavior, 11,* 671 - 684.

[54] Herrmann, D., Raybeck, D., & Gutman, D. (1993). Improving student memory. Seattle, WA: Hogrefe & Huber Publishers

[55] Patanjali (1985). *Integral yoga: The yoga sutras of Patanjali: Translation and commentaries by Sri Swami Sathcidananda. Yogaville*, VA: Integral Yoga Publications. (p. 57).

[56] Jha, A. P., Krompinger, J., & Baime, M. J. (2007). Mindfulness training modifies subsystems of attention. *Cognitive, Affective, & Behavioral Neuroscience, 7,* 109 - 119.

[57] Hanh, T. N. (2008). *The Miracle of Mindfulness: The Classic Guide to Meditation by the world's most*

revered master. New York: Random House.

[58] Lorayne, H. (1990). *How to develop a super power memory.* Hollywood, FL: Fell Publishers. (p. 69)

[59] Minninger, J. & Dugan, E. (1988). *Make your mind work for you: New techniques to improve memory, beat procrastination, increase energy and more!* Emmaus, PA: Rodale Press.

Chapter 5

Associations

"The laws of association govern, in fact, all the trains of our thinking" — William James[1] Speculations about memory go back at least to Plato and Aristotle, who defined the two fundamental poles of opinion on memory. Plato argued that all learning was a kind of remembering, while Aristotle believed our knowledge came from experience. Aristotle proposed we learned by making connections between different sense experiences in accord with certain laws of association. These sense experiences were built up into ideas, which, in turn, could also be associated with each other.

Aristotle is considered the founder of associational psychology and his principles of association remain a core tenet of modern learning theory. He proposed three laws that govern association: the laws of similarity, contrast, and contiguity.[2]

To understand these laws we can watch their operation in the word association test. This test was invented by Darwin's cousin Francis Galton, who used himself as an experimental subject. For his experiment, he drew up a list of 75 words. Once a month for four months he went through the list writing down the first words came to his mind for every item on the list. The four experiments produced

505 associations. Galton was surprised to see that 67% of the associations he generated were repeated at least once. He concluded "this showed much less variety in the mental stock of ideas than I had expected."[3]

Swiss psychiatrist Carl Jung, who carried out his own word association experiments, pointed out the importance of this last point. Since any answer was allowable in word association experiments, one might expect the responses to be random. However, there were patterns in the responses that suggested the operation of Aristotle's laws of association.[4]

The law of similarity says that we associate ideas and experiences that share some resemblance. When asked, in the word association test, to respond to the word "truck" you might say "car." Clearly, cars and trucks share many physical and functional properties.

According to the law of contrast, we tend to associate events that are dramatically different from, or even opposite of, each other. In a word association experiment if asked to respond to the word "white" you are likely to answer "black."

The law of contiguity says that experiences that occur close to each other in time or space will tend to associate together. If asked to respond to word "lightening," you might respond "thunder." These are two events that tend to occur at the same time.

In modern times, a fourth law of association has been proposed, the law of frequency. This law works in conjunction with the law of contiguity. The more times you see two events close together, the stronger the association between them. This law explains learning by repetition. Suppose you wish to learn math facts using flashcards. On one side of the card is written the problem, say 8 * 8 =. On the other side is the answer 64. You learn to associate the information on the two sides of the card because of contiguity. They occur close together in time and space, that is, every time you flip the card over. Because you review the card frequently, this association is made stronger by the law of frequency.[5]

The laws of association are framed in terms of the relationship between ideas, are they similar to each other? Do they occur in the same time or place? But ideas themselves have properties that make them more or less associable. One importance property is strangeness. The stranger, more unusual, an idea the easier it is to form associations with it. This explains what is called the bizarreness effect; bizarre ideas and images are easier to remember than commonplace ones.[6]

Writing in 1886, physician Martin Luther Holbrook gave this example of how we build up associations in our memory. We might learn that the Great Fire of London occurred in 1666. The year 1666 is easily to remember because of the repeating digits. Once we know that fact then it easy to add the fact that there was a plague in London in 1665, one year before 1666 and that the fire played a role in ending the plague. In addition, we could associate the fact that the fire of 1666 gave rise to fire insurance.[7]

Associational psychology was revived in 18th and 19th centuries by a group of British philosophers that included John Locke, David Hume, and John Stuart Mill. A central idea was that our thoughts were build up from the combination of sensations. Using chemistry as a model, each sensation could be thought of as an atom of experience that combined with other such atoms according to the laws of association. Learning here is seen as a kind of mental chemistry with bonds of association forged between elemental sensations to create more complex ideas and concepts

Associationism represents our first science of memory. It was, initially, a purely behavioral science because it made inferences about how memory worked without any understanding of the underlying biological processes. Today we have made some headway in understanding the biology of memory. While our knowledge is incomplete, we now know that associational learning maps onto a process of association between neurons. Thus, associational psychology is very much alive.

We have been using the word association without defining it. Murdock gives us a useful definition: "an association is a rule or relationship between two stored memory traces that maps one into the other."[8] Memories are stored in structural patterns in networks of neurons and these structural patterns are organized by associations. Memory is fundamentally an associative system where information is stored and located based on its relationship to other networked information.[9] William James described it this way:

Each of the associates is a hook to which it hangs a means to fish it up when sunk below the surface. Together they form a network of attachments by which it is woven into the entire tissue of our thought. The secret of a good memory is thus the secret of forming diverse and multiple associations with every fact we retain.[10]

As James says our memory is a network of associations. A network that is continually reorganized by experience. A good way to visualize our memory network is to think of it a mind map similar to those described by Tony Buzan. A mind map is a drawing that represents the connections between ideas we are trying to learn. In a mind map, sometimes called a concept map, ideas are enclosed in circles or ellipses, and the relationships between those ideas are represented by lines.[11] Perhaps, the similarity between mind maps and the actual structure of memory explains why drawing these diagrams does seem to help improve memory.[12]

Another way to understand the associational nature of memory is to examine the words that we store in memory. This aspect of long term memory is called the mental lexicon. While the mental lexicon is not our entire memory network, it is a large and important subset of our long term memory.

We can study the mental lexicon, and by implication the structure of memory itself, by looking at how we remember words. We must be careful here because words are not the same as thoughts. Animals, without language in the human sense, clearly have thoughts in the sense of processing information, possessing cognitive maps, and having felt conscious experience. For humans, however, our thoughts are closely tied to remembered words and the study of how words are efficiently called up from memory must tell us something about how information is stored. The mental lexicon is a vast storehouse of networked words, and we can study the association of information in our brain by studying how we associate words.[13]

In her book, *Words in Mind*, Jean Aitchinson described the words in memory "as linked together in a giant multi-dimensional cobweb, in which every item is attached to scores of others"[14] Today, there is another web, not made by a spider, we can use to understand memory.

A Mind Like Google

In the past the brain and the memories stored in it was said to resemble a library, where information could be located through a system of card catalog organization. Improved technology provided better metaphors. In his popular 1920 book, *The Human Nature Club*, the pioneering educational psychologist Edward Thorndike, described the brain as like "the switchboard in a telegraph office" with "a lot of incoming and outgoing wires and a lot of connecting wires in some central station."[15] This comparison does capture something of the networked structure of our brain. More recently the memory system has been compared to the Internet.

One should be careful with analogies. There are fundamental differences between human memory and the Internet. The Internet stores information in documents that are networked together, while in the brain the information is held in the network connections themselves. As neuroscientist Joaquin Furster pointed out "it is not so much that a memory trace is contained in a network; the memory trace *is* the network."[16]

However, just like the Internet, the structure of human memory is a vast and intricate network of associations. In addition, the process of retrieving information from the brain's network resembles the workings of an Internet search engine. Understanding how a search engine finds information can help us understand our memory.

At its heart the World Wide Web is a set of web pages each with a unique address. The pages are connected to other pages through connections called links. We could draw a diagram of the Web as a set of documents with lines between them. Each line would represent a link. One way to use the web is to enter the address of a website into your browser program. The browser then calls up the page you requested; by clicking on the links on that page you may find other web pages of interest.

Increasingly we have come to rely on the search engine as a way to find information online. We enter a search term and, depending on the availability of the information and the choice of our search terms, we receive a ranked list of web sites that may be relevant to our quest.

How does the search engine find and rank the web pages? First, the search engine finds all the web pages that contain our search terms, then it analyzes the links between the pages. The assumption is that the greater the number of links the more important the information. Sophisticated search engines, like Google, also take into consideration the relative importance of the linking web pages when assigning its rankings. Importance is defined in terms of the number of total links a given web page receives. We can think of the links between pages as associations. The brain and the Internet are both associational networks.

But how similar are these networks? In one experiment, 50 students at Brown University were asked to name the first word that came to mind when shown a cards, each with a single letter of the alphabet. The 21 cards (the letters K, Q, X, Y, and Z were excluded) were shown one at a time. The process was completed twice for each student. We can think of each letter as being like a search term.

For many letters, some responses were more common than others. For example, when given the letter C, 26 students called the word "cat" to mind.

Using a search engine called PageRank, a prototype for the Google search engine, the researchers then queried a database of words drawn from human word association studies. The words in the database were linked together in such a way to represent the frequency of association found in human responses. The ranking of the search engine was remarkably similar to the frequency of responses by the students. For example, just as the word "cat" was the most common response by students shown the letter C, "cat" was also the highest ranked C word by the search engine. Thus, not only is there some resemblance between our memory and the World Wide Web, but, also, between Internet searches and the human memory retrieval.[17]

For human memory we call a search term a cue. A cue is a stimulus that initiates memory retrieval. Any reminder is a cue. William James pointed out how cues were essential for recall. He asked how you would answer if he simply commanded "remember, recollect?" James supplied the obvious response: "what kind of a thing do you wish me to remember?"[18] Clearly some kind of cue is needed because a cue is linked by association to the desired information. A question on an exam, or a hint in a trivia game are examples of cues. Cues include not only external stimuli, but, also, internal stimuli, such as circadian rhythms. For example, getting tired in the evening might remind you to brush your teeth.[19] When your body provides its own cues, we call it state dependent memory.

In state dependent memory our physiological state acts as a cue for memory. There is, for example, a case of a hospitalized man who begins speaking in Welsh while delirious with a fever. He had spoken the language as a child but lost it as he grew older. When he recovered from his fever he again became monolingual.[20] More common examples are cases of individuals, who learn something when drunk, are unable to retrieve the memory when sober, yet succeed in remembering when again intoxicated.

Cues also help explain why we occasionally have difficulty recognizing people. People often change their clothes or hair styles. We may run into people in contexts different from where we usually encounter them. Seeing someone out of context means having fewer cues for memory. We know the clerk every week when we see her at the store, but cannot place her when we meet her at the library. In these cases, we forget because the memory cues are not static.[21]

Harnessing the Power of Associations

Memory is one of the areas where the observations of the ancients still have value for us. No modern person would trust Aristotle's physics. Indeed, the scientific revolution can be said to have begun with Galileo's and Bacon's challenge to the authority of Aristotle. Yet Aristotle's laws of association are still cited in modern psychology texts, and his observations often match the findings of contemporary behavioral psychologists.

Associations may help explain the superior memory of some people with synesthesia. Sherashevsky, the mnemonist studied by Luria, experienced words and sounds as visual images. According to Luria, "once he formed an image, which was always of a particularly vivid nature, it stabilized itself in his memory."[22] Techniques exist to exploit the principles of association to improve our recall. These techniques are called mnemonics, and will be discussed in Chapter 7.

---

[1] James, W. (1890/1950). *The Principles of Psychology*. New York: Dover Publications (p. 88).

[2] Warren, H. C. (1916). Mental associations from Plato to Hume. *Psychological Review, 23*, 208 – 230.

[3] Galton, F. (1883/1951). *Inquiries into human faculty and its development*. London: The Eugenics Society. (p. 138).

[4] Jung, C. G. (1906/1973). The psychopathological significance of the association experiment. In H. Read, et al. (Eds.) *The Collected Works of C. G. Jung*, Vol. 2. (pp. 408 - 425. Princeton, NJ: Princeton University Press.

[5] Powell, R. A., Symbaluk, D. G., & Honey, P. L. (2009). *Introduction to learning and behavior.* 3rd Ed. Belmont, CA: Warsworth.

[6] Dickinson, A. (2007). Learning: The need for a hybrid theory. In H. L. Roediger, Y. Dudai, & S. M. Fizpatrick (Eds.) *Science memory concepts* (pp. 41 - 44). Oxford: Oxford University Press.

[7] Holbrook, M. L. (1886). *How to strengthen the memory; Or, natural and scientific methods of never forgetting.* New York: M. L. Holbrook & Company

[8] Murdock, B. B. (1974). *Human memory: Theory and data.* Potomac, MD: Lawerence Erlbaum Associates.(p. 9).

[9] Fuster, J. M. (1999). *Memory in the cerebral cortex.* Cambridge, MA: MIT Press.

[10] James, W. (1899/1958). *Talks to teachers: On psychology; and to students on some of life's ideals.* New York: W. W. Norton & Company. (p. 90)

[11] Buzan, T. (1984). *Use your head.* London: Guild Publishing.

[12] Farrand, P., Hussain, F., & Hennessy, E. (2002). The efficacy of the mind map study technique. *Medical*

education, 36(5), 426-431.

[13] Aitchison, J. (2003). *Words in the mind: An introduction to the mental lexicon.* Oxford, UK: Blackwell Publishing.

[14] Aitchison, J. (2003). *Words in the mind: An introduction to the mental lexicon.* Oxford, UK: Blackwell Publishing. (p. 84).

[15] Thorndike, E. L. (1920). *The human nature club.* New York: Longmans, Green, and Company. (p. 15).

[16] Fuster, J. M. (1999). *Memory in the cerebral cortex.* Cambridge, MA: MIT Press. (p. 11).

[17] Griffiths, T. L., Steyvers, M., & Firl, A. (2007). Google and the mind: Predicting fluency with Pagerank. *Psychological Science, 18,* 1069 - 1076.

[18] James, W. (1899/1958). *Talks to teachers: On psychology; and to students on some of life's ideals.* New York: W. W. Norton & Company. (p. 87).

[19] Dudai, Y. (2002). *Memory: From A to Z.* Oxford; Oxford University Press.

[20] Quick, R. H. (1888).*How to train the memory: The three A's.* Chicago, IL: E. L. Kellog & Company.

[21] Weinland, J. D. (1957). *How to improve your memory.* New York: Barnes and Noble, Inc.

[22] Luria, A. R. (1968). The mind of a mnemonist: A little book about a vast memory. Cambridge, MA: Harvard University Press. (p. 30)

Chapter 6

Brain Exercise?

The idea of brain exercise is not new. In 1851, the phrenologist O. S. Fowler wrote "I know, indeed, that the brains of most persons become sluggish, almost addled, by thirty, as far as love of study is concerned; and all for want of use. Brain, unexercised, becomes lazy."[1]

Will brain exercise improve your memory? There is now good evidence that brain exercise may be worth the effort. Cognitive engagement, mental activity that is regular and demanding, may protect and improve memory.

In the past, our only evidence for the protective effects of cognitive engagement was anecdotal. It is easy to think of people who remained cognitively engaged through old age. Psychologist James Weinland provided a few examples:

Edison did some of his best work in his seventies. Goethe completed the second part of his *Faust* when over eighty. Victor Hugo died at eighty-three, writing excellent poetry and carrying on unplatonic love affairs to the very end. Titan painted his masterpiece, the "Pietá" at eighty-five. Shaw retained his extraordinary mental alertness until his death at ninety-four.[2]

Yet we are not free to infer from these cases that cognitive engagement prevented senility. These, after all, are anecdotes and could be exceptional cases that do not represent the real pattern. There are, undoubtedly, three pack a day smokers who survive into their eighties, author Kurt Vonnegut was one. Even though Vonnegut lived to an old age, we would not argue that smoking promotes a long life. Nor do we know if cognitive engagement preserved the mental acuity of these individuals or some other factor, perhaps "unplatonic love affairs?"

One reason that anecdotal evidence is unpersuasive is that it is often possible to find counter anecdotes. It is hard to imagine anyone more intellectually engaged than Ralph Waldo Emerson, yet he succumbed to Alzheimer's dementia. [3] Systematic research was needed to decide the question.

One of the most intriguing research projects is known as the Nun Study. In 1991, 678 nuns, all members of the School Sisters of Notre Dame, volunteered to be studied for the rest of their lives. At the beginning of the research, the nuns' ages ranged from 75 to 102 years. They agreed to yearly physical and cognitive examinations and to donate their brains for autopsy upon death. Because the sisters shared a similar lifestyle, environmental variation was reduced. Yet there were substantial differences in cognitive abilities. For example, one sister was debilitated with dementia at age 75, while another lived to be 100 with excellent cognitive skills. [4]

How to account for these differences? In 1930, the nuns had been asked by their religious order to write short autobiographical essays. The essays were found in convent archives making it possible to see if linguistic skill in 1930 predicted cognitive status in the 1990s. It did.

The essays were scored for idea density, a measure of text complexity. Those who showed lower idea density in their writing suffered a higher incidence of Alzheimer's disease.[5] One explanation of this finding is that complex cognitive engagement early in life has a protective effect. But that is not the only possible interpretation. Correlation is not causation, and another possibility might be some genetic factors. After all, the nuns all lived in a similar environment, making heredity a plausible explanation for differences in outcome. In any scientific investigation if one factor is held constant then some other factor must be the cause of differences in the results.

Genes do play a role in intelligence [6] and susceptibility to dementia [7] as do environmental factors. Could it be that smarter people are more resistant to dementia? The nun study cannot settle this question. The environment while similar was not identical for every nun. Nor could researchers control for environmental differences prior to entering the convent.

A study conducted in Sweden tried to control for genetic effects by looking at discordant twin pairs. In the language of behavior genetics, a pair of identical twins are discordant when one twin has a condition and the other does not. Identical twins have the same genes, suggesting that any difference between twins must be environmental in origin. Cases where only one twin has Alzheimer's disease provide important evidence about environmental factors. In this investigation, the researchers identified a number of twin pairs discordant for dementia and looked at occupational differences between affected and unaffected twins. They found that occupations that involved complex work with other people were associated with lower risk of Alzheimer's disease and other types of dementia. This is clear evidence that modifiable environmental factors do play a role in dementia.[8]

We now have good evidence, from controlled randomized experiments, that mental training can reduce the risk of dementia. Psychologist Karlene Ball, of the University of Alabama, and her colleagues conducted such an experiment with 2,832 volunteers in six cities. The volunteers, ages 65 to 94 at the beginning of the study were each assigned randomly to one of four groups. Three of the groups engaged in some kind of mental training, the fourth group served as a control. The mental training consisted of ten sessions over a five to six week period. Each session was 60 to 75 minutes long. Sessions one through five focused on instruction in specific cognitive strategies with opportunities for practice. The final five sessions were solely dedicated to practicing the strategies.

Eleven months later most of the volunteers were given four 75 minute refresher sessions. All three forms of cognitive training, focused on memory, reasoning or speed of processing, were shown to have positive effects. At the end of the study volunteers showed real improvement in the skills they were trained. In the words of the study's authors "a significant segment of trained individuals went forward through 2 years of life with better cognitive skills than did the controls."[9] The message is clear:

cognitive engagement affords some protection against dementia, and deliberate mental training can confer real benefits.

It has been suggested that the rising tide of Alzheimer's disease may be a consequence of our modern failure to provide our memories with adequate exercise. Since we rely so much on external memory storage, we allow our brain's memory to become flabby and weak. As David Shenk, author of the book *The Forgetting: Alzheimer's: Portrait of an Epidemic,* put it, "not doing the mental work means not building those internal connections between neurons."[10] We do physical exercise to maintain health in an environment where most occupations no longer demand muscular exertion. In a similar sense, we may need mental exercise to counteract the effects of a less demanding cognitive environment.

What type of cognitive training is best? Some caution is in order. We should be aware that many of the claims made for commercial cognitive enhancement programs have never been verified.[11] The best advice we can give is to choose learning tasks that are both challenging and interesting. Learning a new language would be a good candidate activity. A study of Alzheimer's patients in Toronto compared those who were bilinguals with those who spoke only one language. On average, bilinguals showed fewer dementia symptoms four years later than monolinguals. In addition, once diagnosed with dementia, bilinguals has slower rates of cognitive decline.[12] The study had some limitations, for example, there is an element of subjectivity in determining the onset of dementia. Also, the study was correlational; while it does show us that bilingualism is associated with protection from dementia, it cannot prove it is the cause. For example, it is possible that bilingualism is a proxy for some other variable, perhaps some cultural or dietary practice that might be the real source of the protection. On the other hand, the protective effect of language learning is certainly a plausible explanation. Given our limited knowledge, learning a new language seems worth trying. It is hard to imagine any harm and at minimum one would gain the benefit of learning a new language.

Taking classes, through universities, community colleges, or adult education programs, would also be excellent choices. The ongoing structure of a class that meets at regular intervals can motivate you to persist in your efforts. Try new things, choose classes that will deepen your skills or introduce you to something new. Become an enthusiastic novice. Laugh off the inevitable mistakes that every beginner makes and try again. Perhaps this is what the Zen Buddhists mean when they tell us "the goal of practice is always to keep our beginner's mind."[13]

Challenge Yourself with Discrepant Information

There is some emerging evidence that suggests that we receive the greatest cognitive benefit from being exposed to discrepant information, facts and opinions that challenge us to alter our perspective.[14] There is a strong bias for us to seek out only the information that confirms our current beliefs. This is called confirmation bias. Not only do we seek out information in accord with current world view, we ignore or reject information that challenges our assumptions.[15] We often do this by employing the *ad hominem* fallacy, when someone says something that we disagree with we dismiss that person as being ignorant or evil. We conclude that any argument made be a person so benighted must be wrong. Logicians point out that it is inappropriate to infer the truth of an argument based on some characteristic of the person making the arguments. All arguments must stand and fall on evidence and logic.

It is healthy to assume that for almost every belief that we have there is someone who is smarter and better intentioned than ourselves who holds a different point of view. The point is not that all of our current opinions are wrong, only that we should be open to the possibility that some of our opinions may be in error or at least in need of revision. If we never listen to people with different opinions, we are in danger of stagnating in our certitude. "The unexamined life is not worth living"[16] and examination means critical self scrutiny, thus we should seek out opportunities to listen to intelligent and thoughtful people from different points of view and not be afraid to engage them in dialogue. Today this is very easy to do with such websites as TED, Bloggingheads.tv, and FORA.TV.

When we begin to learn something new we tend to prefer to receive positive feedback about our performance. As we become more expert our preference tends to shift towards more critical feedback. This may be because beginners almost always have lower levels of performance and may find excessively critical feedback discouraging. But as we become more expert, and our performance improves, critical evaluations of our performance becomes more informative. Thus, expert performers become more attentive to critical feedback and use this information a the basis for continued improvement.[17] We need not fear, nor should we be discouraged by, critical feedback.

Physical Exercise

While mental exercise is central to the memory improvement advocated in this book, good physical health also contributes to a better memory. There is important evidence that regular physical exercise improves memory and increases resistance to dementia.

One study of adults between the ages of 55 and 80, found that an exercise program of 40 minutes of vigorous walking there days a week led to a 2% increase in the size of the hippocampus, a brain structure crucial to memory, and improved performance on a test of spatial memory. These results were particularly significant since the hippocampus tends to shrink with age.[18]

I believe that it is possible to integrate both physical and mental exercise into a comprehensive program of memory improvement. Every morning I walk for an hour either outside or on my treadmill. I use this walking time to study languages using mp3 language programs such as Pimsleur and to listen to podcasts, such as the Slate Political Gabfest

(http://www.slate.com/articles/podcasts/gabfest.html)   or
The Partially Examined Life (http://www.partially
examinedlife.com/). Time to get moving!

Diet

Healthy diet should also play a role in your memory
improvement plan. I am not a nutritionist, but I am
very impressed with the work of physician Neal
Barnard and enthusiastically recommend his book
Power Foods for the Brain. This popular book is well
ground in the available science and is a good starting
point for understanding how diet can prevent
memory loss[19]

[1] Fowler, O. S. (1851). *Memory and intellectual
improvement applied to self-education and juvenile
instruction.* New York: Fowlers and Wells. (p. 183).

[2] Weinland, J. D. (1957). *How to improve your memory.*
New York: Barnes and Noble, Inc. (p. 32).

[3] Shenk, D. (2003). *The forgetting: Alzheimer's:
Portrait of an epidemic.* New York: Anchor Books.

[4] Snowdon, D. A. (2003). Healthy aging and dementia:
Findings from the nun study. *Annals of Internal
Medicine, 5,* 450 - 454.

[5] Snowdon, D. A., Greiner, W. R., & Markesbery, W. R.
(2000). Linguistic Ability in Early Life and the
Neuropathology of Alzheimer's Disease and
Cerebrovascular Disease: Findings from the Nun
Study. *Annals of the New York Academy of Sciences,
903,* 34 - 38.

[6] Nisbett, R. E. et al (2012). Intelligence: New findings and theoretical developments. *American Psychologist, 67,* 130 - 159.

[7] Pollen, D. A. (1996). *Hannah's heirs: The quest for the genetic origins of Alzheimer's disease.* New York: Oxford University Press.

[8] Andel, R. et al. (2005). Complexity of work and risk of Alzheimer's disease: A population based study of Swedish twins. *Journal of Gerontology, 60B,* 251 - 258.

[9] Ball, K. et al(2002). Effects of cognitive training interventions with older adults: A randomized controlled trial. *JAMA, 288,* 2271–2281. (p. 2281).

[10] Shenk, D. (2003). *The forgetting: Alzheimer's: Portrait of an epidemic.* New York: Anchor Books. (p. 233).

[11] Papp, K. V., Stephen, J. W., & Snyder, P. J., (2009). Immediate and delayed effects of cognitive interventions in healthy elderly: A review of current literature and future directions. *Alzheimer's & Dementia, 5,* 50 - 60.

[12] Bialystok, E., Craik, F. I. M., & Freedman, M. (2007). Bilingualism as a protection against the onset of dementia. *Neuropsychologica, 45,* 459 - 464.

[13] Suzuki, S. (1970). *Zen mind, beginner's mind.* New York: Weatherhill. (p. 17).

[14] Furnham, A., & Ribchester, T. (1995). Tolerance of ambiguity: A review of the concept, its measurement

and applications. Current Psychology, 14(3), 179-199.

[15] Nickerson, R. S. (1998). Confirmation bias: A ubiquitous phenomenon in many guises. Review of general psychology, 2(2), 175.

[16] Plato (1895). *A selection of passages from Plato for English readers from the translation by B. Jowett.* Oxford: Clarendon press. (p. 107).

[17] Finkelstein, S. R., & Fishbach, A. (2012). Tell me what I did wrong: Experts seek and respond to negative feedback. *Journal of Consumer Research, 39, 22 - 38.*

[18] Erickson, E. et al. (2011). Exercise training increases size of hippocampus and improves memory. *PNAS, 108, 3017 - 3022.*

[19] Barnard, N. (2013). *Power Foods for the Brain: An Effective 3-step Plan to Protect Your Mind and Strengthen Your Memory.* New York: Hachette Digital, Inc.

Chapter 7
Mnemonics

How did Akira Haraguchi memorize 100,000 digits of pi? He used mnemonics.

Psychologist Francis Bellezza defined mnemonics as "special methods of memorizing that ensure that large amounts of information can be remembered for a relatively long time."[1] Mnemonics employ the principles of association. Typically, a mnemonic requires us to create an artificial association between something easily remembered and information that is hard to remember. Once the link is forged we are able to hold the desired information securely in memory.[2]

Everyone has some experience with mnemonics. For example, you may remember the order of operation in algebra by recalling the phrase "please excuse my dear aunt Sally." The first letter of each word standing for a specific operation: parentheses, exponentiation, multiplication, division, addition and subtraction.

Mnemonics have often been dismissed by psychologists and educators as tricks of little value. No less an authority than William James described their use as "poor, trivial, and silly."[3] James' hostility seems to have set the stage for decades of opposition to the use of mnemonics. In 1944, Medical librarian Julian Scherr, writing in the *Elementary School Journal*, lamented that teachers "violently oppose"[4] the teaching of mnemonic systems.

This opposition, violent or otherwise, has been characterized as mnemophobia and is a common prejudice among educators. Jan Hulstijn, an expert on second language learning, wondered why language teachers did not use highly effective mnemonic methods in their instruction. He found that teachers and textbook authors either did not know about these techniques or thought of them as "unnatural."[5]

Mnemonics *are* unnatural in the sense that they are consciously created associations manufactured for the specific purpose of enhancing our memory. Rather than depend upon natural associations, we use our knowledge of the principles of association to make information more memorable. Perhaps it is best to think of mnemonics as "manufactured synethesia."[6] You will recall that the automatic association between senses, such as sound and color, experienced by people with synesthesia seems to have a memory enhancing effect. What we do with mnemonics is to create an association that makes material memorable. Often our goal is to create a vivid visual image for information that is not visual. In one of his memory books, Harry Lorayne tells us "you'll learn how to make everything *visual,* including what you hear." Later, in the same book, he says "applying my systems will enable you to see the names you hear!"[7]

People are primates and primates are visually dominant animals. Your dog has a much better sense of smell than you, but, chances are, you see better than your dog. We devote a large area of the brain to processing visual information. Notice our problem remembering names. We often recognize the face, a visual recognition task that is generally easy for people, but, we cannot remember the name. Remembering a name is a verbal recall task that is much more difficult. A standard memory trick to remember names is to create some image that links the person's physical appearance with the name. Harry Lorayne gives this example of trying to learn the name of a Ms. Van Nuys, a woman with prominent eyes: "I would see moving vans driving out of Miss Van Nuys' eyes and making terribly loud noises. So loud that you have to hold your ears."[8] Lorayne emphasizes that it is important to create a distinctive exaggerated image involving more than one sense, in this case sight and sound. What Lorayne has done here is to create artificial synesthesia. These associations are often unflattering, and you would be wise not to share them with others. They are, however, quite effective.

Mnemonics also impose an artificial organization. Organized information is easier to remember than unorganized information. For example, it is easier to remember the names of the Apollo 11 astronauts if we notice that their names can be arranged in pseudo-alphabetical order: Neil **A**rmstrong, **B**uzz Aldrin, and Michael **C**ollins. Organization is a kind of binding together, it allows us to treat a number of separate facts as if they were a unit. In addition, when information is organized together it is easier to find meaning in it. That is, it is easier to make connections between the new information and information already stored in long term memory.

The utility and effectiveness of mnemonics are undeniable. If I ask you how many days are there in April, there is a good chance that you would resort to the mnemonic poem: "Thirty days has September." So, even if you think you despise mnemonics, you probably use them. Indeed, the spontaneous use of mnemonics by students is common.[9]

According to psychologist A. Charles Catania "Educational systems have tended to emphasize learning through understanding and have correspondingly de-emphasized or even discouraged memorization. It's unlikely, however, that a learner will be disadvantaged by learning in more than one way, so mnemonics can be effective supplements to other methods of study."[10]

There is now a substantial body of work showing that mnemonics are useful tools for improving memory; they do not have the harmful consequences imputed by William James. For example, we have evidence that students who spontaneously used mnemonics have higher GPAs than those who do not.[11] In addition, training in mnemonics has been shown to help older people with declining memories.[12]

Another area where mnemonics have been shown to be effective is learning foreign language vocabularies. Researchers, teachers, and students identify learning vocabulary as the most difficult part of mastering a new language. Native speakers are more likely to understand someone with poor grammar skills but adequate vocabulary than someone who knows the rules of correct grammar but lacks the needed words[13]

The keyword method for foreign language vocabulary involves finding an English word or phrase that sounds like the foreign word and then making an association between the two words. In the keyword method two mnemonic associations are made, first an acoustic link between the sound of the foreign word and the sound of the English word. Then an imagery link is created that connects the two words.[14] For example, the Russian word for throat is *garlo*. *Garlo* sounds like gargle, an activity carried out in the throat. It is easy to form a visual image to cement this association.[15] Michael Gruneberg has created courses for over a dozen languages using the keyword method. He markets these courses at www.linkwordlanguages.com.

The keyword method is a kind of scaffolding that supports performance during early language learning. Over time the student learns to make a direct association between the word and its meaning and reliance on the mnemonic fades away.

Are students better off creating their own keywords or should they use ones provided by the instructor? Experimental research found that while student created keywords worked better than not using the keyword method, student performance was better when using instructor provided keywords. One possible reason for this that not all keywords are equally effective, some associations may be more difficult to form than others. Research and experience may produce lists of highly effective keywords. Rather than letting students stumble on the keyword method by accident, keywords should be explicitly taught as part of the curriculum.[16]

Mnemonics also improve higher order thinking skills. As noted before, memory is a prerequisite for efficient higher order processing. Russell Carney and

Joel Levin, two educational physiologists, who have conducted decades of research on mnemonics, found that "by cementing lower-order connections, mnemonic strategies have produced higher-order learning benefits both in their own right and in conjunction with formal information-organizing structures, such as matrices and taxonomies."[17]

Why are mnemonics effective? Carney and Levin, identified the three Rs of mnemonics: recoding, relating, and retrieving in this example:

> First, an unfamiliar term is recoded to make it more concrete and visualizable (e.g. nefasch became knee). Second, the associated terms are related by way of a compound visual image or picture (the image of a knee pressing down on the fish's snout). Finally, retrieval is accomplished by retracing the retrieval path established by the technique.[18]

Mnemonics make information more memorable. For example, we might take a difficult to remember vocabulary term and recoded it as a visual image. Concrete visual images are often more memorable than abstract unfamiliar words. Recently I was listening to a podcast while working out. In the course of the program a philosopher, Derek Parfit was mentioned. I was not familiar with Parfit's work and decided to read up on him. But here was my problem, wearing my sweat-clothes and a mile from home I couldn't write down his name. I had to rely on my memory. So I created a visual image, an oil derrick sitting on an ice cream parfait, spewing ice cream out of its top. I was able to remember his name with ease. I should mention that in writing this account I came across the interesting fact that the oil derrick gets its name from Thomas Derrick an Elizabethan executioner who invented a type of gallows (I verified this in the Oxford English Dictionary).

There is a critical shortage of good mnemonics, and the good ones that do exist are not well known. When I ask my students to give examples of mnemonics, they often only know a few very popular ones such as HOMES for remembering the names of the Great Lakes (Huron, Ontario, Michigan, Erie, and Superior). There are some good collections of mnemonics available. Some of the best are for medical students faced with the task of learning human anatomy. A good example is Stephen Goldberg's *Clinical Anatomy Made Ridiculously Simple*.[19] Others, such as *Every Good Boy Deserves Fudge* by Rod Evans,[20] and *i before e (except after c)* by Judy Parkinson,[21] provide more general examples. These books suggest that mnemonics could be extended to help in a much larger range of learning tasks.

First Letter Mnemonics

Which is the bad cholesterol? Is it LDL or HDL? Easy! The bad cholesterol is the Lousy (**LDL**) one, and HDL is **Healthy**.[22]

For students, the most widely used type of mnemonic is the first letter mnemonic, also called the acronym method.[23] where a word, sentence, phrase or poem is committed to memory and the first letter of each word serves as a cue for the information. The HOMES mnemonic and "please excuse my dear aunt Sally" are both examples of the first letter mnemonics.

You might remember the three great Greek philosophers, Socrates, Plato, and Aristotle, in order of their birth with the acronym SPA.[24]

Students will often be called on to memorize material for which there are no available mnemonics. This demands creativity on the part of the student. Sometimes the first letters can be arranged into a word, such as WISE to remember the British Isles (Wales, Ireland, Scotland, England), more often it will require the creation of some memorable phrase.[25] For example, here is a first letter mnemonic for the potentially useful task of learning the Dewey Decimal System:

Generally, philosophical religionists see language scientifically to favor literary history.

Category	Catalog Number	Mnemonic
General Works	0	Generally
Philosophy and psychology	100	philosophical
religion	200	religionists
Social Science	300	see
Language	400	language
Science	500	scientifically
Technology	600	to
Fine arts	700	favor
Literature	800	literary
History	900	history

Adapted from Evans[26]

One interesting feature of mnemonics is that they

often fall away as the target information becomes well learned.[27] Indeed, you sometimes discover that you have to rely on the target information to remember the mnemonic. I have had that experience with the Dewey Decimal mnemonic; I now know the Dewey system well enough that I use it to recall the mnemonic rather than using the mnemonic to recover the information. One can get a sense of what this feels like from the world's most useless mnemonic, one to remember the names of the digits from one to ten, "Only The Truly Forgetful Fellow Should Summon Each Number Thusly." The first letter of each word corresponding to the first letter of each digit. The only way I can remember this mnemonic is by referring back to the numbers. In effect, the numbers one to ten are the mnemonic device to remember the mnemonic.

On the other hand when the material is used infrequently the mnemonic can be like an old friend available to help when needed. Occasionally, I have need to recall the basic trigonometric functions and would be lost without the word SOHCAHTOA that encodes the needed information (**S**in = **O**pposite / **H**ypotenuse, **C**os = **A**djacent / **H**ypotenuse, **T**an = **O**pposite / **A**djacent).

The examples given so far are all single purpose mnemonics, each one codes a small specific set of information, but, as Bellezza points out, first letter mnemonics have limitations. For example, if the list of material is too long it may be hard to use this approach, or if many of the items you have to learn start with the same letter.[28] In addition, it is not a helpful approach for remembering numbers as the

PIN for your ATM.

Fortunately, there are other generalized mnemonic strategies that can be applied to a wider range of material.

Length of Word Mnemonics

A length of word mnemonic is used to remember some important number. The length of each word in a verse or memorable phrase encodes the sequential digits. For example, one mnemonic for pi to four places is "may I draw a circle" (3.1415).[29] Another, "How I need a drink alcoholic in nature, after the heavy lectures involving quantum mechanics" encodes the value of pi, 3.14159265358979, out to 14 places.[30]

Link Method

One example of a generalized mnemonic technique is the link system where a list of material can be linked together by connecting each item to the next, usually using some vivid visual image. An example of this technique can be found in *Yo, Millard Fillmore!* This delightful book helps children learn the names of the American Presidents in order of their terms in office.

For example, everyone knows that Washington is the first President, so imagine a giant washing machine sitting in front of the white house washing a ton of laundry. Now imagine that you open the washing machine up and inside you see large atoms being in the laundry tub. Now you have the name of the second president, Adams. Each president's name is imagined in some bizarre or silly image, and these images are linked together.[31]

The Russian mnemonist Sherashevsky used a form of the link method when Luria asked him to remember a long and complicated algebra formula. The formula began

$$N \cdot \sqrt{}$$

Sherashevsky created a story that mapped on to the symbols in the equation. It began, "Neiman (N) came out and jabbed at the ground with his cane (.). He looked up at a tall tree which resembled the square-root sign ($\sqrt{}$)."[32]

Number Peg Method

In the peg method, sometimes called the minor peg system, an individual memorizes a fixed set of ordered mnemonic cues.[33] It can be used to learn ordered and unordered lists, such as a set of historical events or your weekly shopping. The technique relies on the use of vivid visual images.

The most widely used peg system is the number peg method. This system invented by John Sambrook in 1889 and a simplified version is described in most books on memory improvement.[34] The peg word system is easy to learn and can supplement other mnemonic devices we will be learning, such as the Dominic system. The first step is to create a numbered list of ten mnemonics pegs. Each peg word should rhymes with its respective number making the list easier to learn. Here is a suggested list, but you should modify if you can think of words that are more memorable to you. For example, if the word "bricks" is easier for you to visualize than the word "sticks," by all means, use it as your peg word for number six.

Number	Peg Word
1	Gun
2	Shoe
3	Tree
4	Door
5	Hive
6	Sticks
7	Heaven
8	Gate
9	Vine
10	Hen

Once you have committed the list to memory, you are now ready to try to learn a list. What you will do is to make a vivid visual association with each item. So let's try to learn a grocery list. Suppose you want to purchase the following ten items:

1. oatmeal, 2. apples, 3. bananas, 4. spaghetti, 5. peanut butter, 6. carrots, 7. mushrooms, 8. maple syrup, 9. baked beans, 10. soy milk.

On the following page is a chart suggesting visual associations between the items and the peg words.

Number	Peg Word	Item	Association
1	Gun	Oatmeal	Gun shooting out oatmeal (instead of bullets)
2	Shoe	Apples	Shoe crushing apples under its heel
3	Tree	Bananas	A tree with bananas hanging on it
4	Door	Spaghetti	Spaghetti forcing itself through a door
5	Hive	peanut butter	Beehive made of peanut butter
6	Sticks	Carrots	A bundle of carrots wrapped up like sticks
7	Heaven	Mushrooms	Giant mushrooms growing in heaven
8	Gate	Maple syrup	A gate holding back a flood of maple syrup
9	Vine	Baked Beans	Cans of baked beans growing on a vine
10	Hen	Soy milk	A hen laying a carton of soy milk

If some of these associations seem bizarre, so much the better. The more bizarre, the easier to remember, a phenomenon called the bizarreness effect. It is important to try to create vivid visual images for each association. If, in addition, you can link the image to something you already know, the easier it will be to remember. For example, when I think of a gate holding back a flood of maple syrup, I am reminded of the Boston Molasses Disaster of 1919 (this really happened, look it up).

Some have worried that reusing the same pegs might interfere with the learning of subsequent lists. However, research suggests that the number peg system can be used over and over again.[35]

The Alphabet Peg System

For memorizing longer lists many books propose the use of an alphabet peg system where each letter of the alphabet is associated with a visual image. For example, A is associated with the image of an ape, and B is associated with the image of a bee.

However, there may be problems that make the alphabet peg system more difficult to use than the numeric peg system. The alphabet peg system may create greater interference and weaker associations than the number peg system. While we generally don't associate words with the digits 0 — 9, we do associate many words with the letters of the alphabet. How many A to Z alphabet books did you read as a child or have read to your children? Should A be an ape or apple? While the numeric peg system has a simple rhyming rule for associating numbers with words, such as one with gun it is harder to make such associations with the alphabet. Tony Buzan suggests, when possible, to use words that sound identical to the letter, such as "sea" for C and "bee" for B.[36] But this rule can only be applied to some letters. Morris Young and Walter Gibson also acknowledge problems and propose that the list be learned as a linked chain of objects. So that A is represented as an arrow being shot at a bird that represents B. The bird is running away from a cat who represents C and so on.[37] However, given the complexity of the system it is probably not worth the effort to learn alphabetic peg system. The method of loci, the technique used by the ancients, is a better approach for longer lists.

The Method of Loci

The method of loci, also called the journey method or the topical system, is a form of the peg method. Here, however, each peg is a geographic location arranged in a sequence where one imagines a well rehearsed trip from one location to the next. Each location in the sequence serves as a mnemonic peg.

The invention of this system is credited to the Greek poet Simonides around 500 BC. According to the legend Scopas, a nobleman and the winner of an Olympic game, hired Simonides to compose and recite a poem at a victory banquet. While the poem composed and recited by Simonides glorified the athlete, it included praise for the twin gods Castor and Pollux. These two deities were traditionally associated with sport, but Scopas was displeased that they were mentioned in the poem. He felt he should not have to share his glory with others, and he refused to pay Simonides.

While Scopas and Simonides were arguing, a messenger arrived and insisted Simonides see two men waiting outside for him. When Simonides left the banquet hall, the building collapsed killing all inside.

When the relatives of the dead arrived, they found

the bodies were so crushed and mutilated that they could not identify them. Simonides, however, recreated the banquet hall in his mind. Moving from place to place in his mind's eye, he was able to name or describe each individual at each location in the building.[38] This imaginary moving from place to place making an association at each point in the mental journey became the basis for the traditional memory systems of ancient times. This system was so widely used it has even affected our language giving rise to the phrases "in the first place," "in the second place" and the word "topic," which comes from the Greek word for place.

Think about some building or place that you are intimately familiar with, perhaps your home or the building where you work. Imagine yourself walking up to the building opening the front door and making a tour of all the rooms. For most of us, it is very easy to call up a visual image of a highly familiar place and imagine a journey through it. In the journey method we designate certain points on the route as pegs to associate information.

Humans are very good at processing spatial information, and this seems to explain the effectiveness of the journey method.[39] Indeed, there is evidence that some neurons in the brain's hippocampus, the structure essential for forming long term memories, are specialized for spatial information.[40]

The journey method requires us to construct a journey in our mind where one location follows another in sequence from beginning to end. The journey can be a real or imagined place. The longer the journey, the more information we can accommodate. In the past memorists would often use, or imagine, palaces for their mental journeys, because they were large with memorable locations. Because of this, the buildings that we construct or reconstruct in our minds have come to be called memory palaces

At Home with the Three Bears

A good choice for your first memory palace might be your childhood home, of which you are likely to have a good memory. However, since I do not know the layout of your family's estate let's, for the purpose of illustration, construct a memory palace from a popular children's story that contains some location information, "Goldilocks and the Three Bears." The story was originally written by British Poet Robert Southey, perhaps drawn from earlier folklore, but most of know the adaptation written by Joseph Cundall.[41]

Imagine the story from the point that Goldilocks arrives at the bears' cottage. Imagine what the cottage looks like and create in your mind a picture of the front door. As Goldilocks walks through the door, she enters into the kitchen where she sees three bowls of porridge. She tries the first big bowl and finds it too hot, she tries the second somewhat smaller bowl of porridge and finds it too cold. The final smallest bowl is just right, and she eats it all. You, of course, know the rest of the story, but we can draw up a table of sequential locations and events each one acting as a memory hook:

1. Goldilocks at the door to the bear's cottage
2. Goldilocks in the kitchen
3. She tries the big bowl of porridge and finds it too hot
4. She tries the middle bowl of porridge and finds it too cold
5. She tries the small bowl of porridge and finding it just right, sl eats it
6. She enters the living room
7. She tries the big chair, but it is too high for her
8. She tries the middle chair, but it is too wide for her
9. She tires the small chair, it is just right, but it breaks under he weight
10. She enters the bedroom
11. She tries the big bed, but it is too hard
12. She tries the middle bed, but it is too soft
13. She tries the small bed, and it is just right, she falls asleep

In order to use the journey you would first rehearse the story in your mind creating a vivid mental image of each step in Goldilocks' travel through the bears' cottage. Then you would make a vivid visual association between each stage of the journey and the item you want to memorize.

We saw how Solomon Shereshevsky used something akin to the journey method. His synesthesia allowed him to create vivid images and associate them with points along a trip. As Foer notes what we do with mnemonics is a kind of "manufactured synesthesia."[42] So it is important that you make your images as vivid as possible to capture this synesthesia like effect.

Let's see if we can use this journey to learn the

names of the 12 signs of the zodiac. Remember to make the image as vivid as possible, imagine colors, sounds and actions.

1. Goldilocks at the door to the bear's cottage. Imagine the door is guarded by Aries, a giant ram
2. Goldilocks in the kitchen. Imagine Taurus the bull, knocking down china from the kitchen shelves
3. She tries the big bowl of porridge and finds it too hot. Gemini, the twins, are fighting over who has to eat the hot porridge. "You eat it!" "No you eat it!"
4. She tries the middle bowl of porridge and finds it too cold. Crawling out of the cold porridge is Cancer, the crab. Imagine the crab wearing earmuffs and a scarf.
5. She discovers Leo the lion, contented, happily eating the just right bowl of porridge
6. She enters the living room. An attractive young woman, Virgo, the virgin, stands at the doorway to the living room
7. Goldilocks tries the big chair, but it is too high for her. Balanced on the very high chair is a set of scales the symbol for Libra
8. She tries the middle chair, but it is too wide for her. In the middle chair imagine the menacing scorpion, Scorpio. Remember to make each image as visual and memorable as possible. For example, you might think of Scorpio being bright red.
9. She tires the small chair, it is just right, but it breaks under her weight. Sagittarius, the archer, half man, half-horse. Standing on the chair causes it to break because of his massive weight

10. She enters the bedroom: At the door to the bedroom Capricorn, a goat.
11. She tries the big bed, but it is too hard. Imagine Aquar the water bearer trying to sleep on the hard bed and spilli water all over it from his water jug
12. She tries the middle bed, but it is too soft. Imagine Pisc the giant fish, floundering in the too soft bed.
13. She tries the small bed, and it is just right, she falls asle There are only twelve signs so we don't need this step.

There is, perhaps, some irony in having to use the method of loci to teach the zodiac signs. In antiquity, the signs and order of the zodiac were so well known, that it was often used as a memory palace.

One advantage of the method of loci is that you can take the journey in either direction. For example, you could start with Pisces the fish flopping in the too soft bed and work your way back to Aries at the front door. You would have trouble trying to do this with the alphabet peg method since most of us have trouble reciting the alphabet in reverse order. Our human ability to reason spatially makes reversing the journey easy.

In their excellent book, *Mindhacker*, Ron Hale-Evans and Marty Hale-Evans recommend using well practiced video games and role playing games for constructing a memory journey.[43] A version of the journey method was once widely practiced in schools for many years where students imagine a journey through countries being studied in geography. The countries are studied in the order they would occur in an actual journey. The idea of this teaching procedure is to help the students engage their imaginative faculties, and, thus, better remember the material.

Phonetic Alphabets

There are several mnemonic systems for remembering sequences of numbers such as dates, phone numbers or mathematical constants, all based on the principle of associating each digit with a letter. A string of digits is translated into a string of letters and those letters are turned into memorable words or names. These can be easily stored in memory and translated back into numbers when needed. These systems, called phonetic alphabets or analytic substitutions, have a long history. According to Morris Young, the system was first proposed in its modern form by the French mathematician Pietro Herigon in 1634.[44]

Over the centuries many different phonetic alphabets have been devised. The most widely used is called the major system, based on a set of associations between consonant sounds and numbers. However, I recommend the one devised by Dominic O'Brien, who won the world memory championship eight times. In May of 2002 he memorized 54 packs of playing cards, 2008 cards in total, shuffled together. He recalled the entire series in order with only eight errors.[45] O'Brien is clear that his native memory ability is quite ordinary and that he relies on learned memory strategies.[46]

His approach, called the Dominic system, appears to be an improved version of one proposed by George Crowther in 1870.[47] Besides being O'Brien's first name Dominic is also an acronym for the systems basic principle: **D**ecipherment of **M**nemonically **I**nterpreted **N**umbers into **C**haracters. O'Brien assigns different letters to the digits zero to nine, according to this scheme:

1	A
2	B
3	C
4	D
5	E
6	S
7	G
8	H
9	N
0	O

O'Brien describes his system as "'seeing' numbers as images."[48] For example, using these digits one can remember number pairs by associating then with the initials of people, historical figures, celebrities, or personal acquaintances. Suppose you wanted to remember that you are staying in hotel room 32, in the Dominic system this maps onto the letters CB, which you might associate with the comic strip character Charlie Brown. You could imagine opening your hotel room door and being surprised to see Charlie Brown there.

I use the Dominic system to remember the value of absolute zero on the Celsius scale, I constructed the phrase "Billy Graham, Cold," which I remember by creating a vivid image of the preacher Billy Graham sitting on an ice cube. In the Dominic system Billy Graham represents 27 and C, the first letter of the word Cold, stands for 3. I know that absolute zero is very cold so it must be a negative value. Thus, I remember that the Celsius temperature for absolute zero is -273 degrees.

To remember the number of feet in a mile, I created the word EBHO, which encodes the number 5,280.

We can extend the Dominic system to remember long strings of digits such as the number Pi. The first few digits of Pi are 3.1415926535. We could assume that you know the first digit is 3, but if you don't you could use the number peg system. Think of the symbol for pi, π, as the trunk of a tree. In the peg system, tree means number 3. Now let's makeup a story where each character's name codes two digits in the Dominic system. Political activist Angela Davis (14) is giving a speech. If Angela Davis doesn't conjure up a vivid image for you, perhaps, you might be able to use Albus Dumbledore from the Harry Potter stories. Albert Einstein (15), who was in the audience, leaves the speech, perhaps riding his bicycle. Where does he go? To the nude beach (92)! What occurs at such a beach? Sex education (65)! Who teaches the class? Must be someone sexy, like Clint Eastwood (35). Now we have created a set of vivid images arranged in an easy to remember story. Run through the story again, and you will see how easy it is to remember an otherwise meaningless sequence of digits.

Mnemonics and Creativity

One point should be clear. While mnemonics have been dismissed as rote or mechanical they actually involve the harnessing of creativity in service of memory. Tony Buzan, author of many popular memory improvement books, points out that the act of association involved in mnemonics is profoundly creative.[49]

The Limitations of Mnemonics

Mnemonics constitute a powerful memory improvement technology. Unfortunately, mnemonics cannot be applied to all situations, and mnemonics do have limitations of which we need to be aware. For example, the keyword method of learning foreign language vocabulary works best for words that physical objects that we can easily visualize. In addition, not all words lend themselves to the keyword approach.[50]

While techniques like the Dominic phonetic alphabet system are powerful, many people do not have a pressing need to remember long series of numbers.[51] This may explain why people are often disappointed with memory improvement courses. While the techniques do work — they often do not seem very useful to the real world memory issues that most of us face. Joshua Foer in his entertaining and informative book on his successful attempt to win the U.S. Memory Championship details the complex mnemonic system he had to master. Foer reports that the mnemonic systems do help him with certain types of real world memory tasks. However, he notes "any information that couldn't be neatly converted into an image and dropped into a memory palace was just as hard for me to retain as it always had been."[52]

Fortunately, other techniques exist for improving memory. While mnemonics have been used for centuries, there are newer, more powerful techniques that grow out of modern memory science. For our purposes, the most important insights come from research that began with the memory experiments of Herman Ebbinghaus.

[1] Bellezza, F. S. (1981). Mnemonic devices: Classification, characteristics, and criteria. *Review of Educational Research, 51*, 247 - 275. (p. 1).

[2] Fauvel-Gouruad, F. (1845). Phreno-mnemotechny; Or, the art of memory. New York: Wiley and Putnam.

[3] James, W. (1899/1958). *Talks to teachers: On psychology; and to students on some of life's ideals.* New York: W. W. Norton & Company. (p. 93).

[4] Scherr. J. M. (1944). Simple memory devices for the classroom. *The Elementary School Journal, 45*, 225 - 230. (p. 227).

[5] Hulstijn, J. H. (1997). Mnemonic methods in foreign language vocabulary learning: Theoretical considerations and pedagogical implications. In J. Coady & T. Huckin (Eds.). *Second language vocabulary acquisition: A rationale for pedagogy.* (pp. 203 - 224). Cambridge, UK: Cambridge

University Press. (p. 210).

[6] Foer, J., (2011). *Moonwalking with Einstein, The art and science of remembering everything.* New York: The Penguin Press. (p. 44).

[7] Lorayne, H. (1975). *Remembering people: The key to success.* New York: Warner Books. (p. 20, pp. 24 - 25).

[8] Lorayne, H. (1990). *How to develop a super power memory.* Hollywood, FL: Fell Publishers. (p. 145)

[9] Carlson, R. F., Kincaid, J. P., Lance, S., & Hodgson, T. (1976). Spontaneous use of mnemonic and grade point average. *The Journal of Psychology, 92,* 117 - 122.

[10] Catania, A. C. (1998). *Learning* (4th edition). Upper Saddle River, NJ: Prentice Hall. (p. 323).

[11] Carlson, R. F., Kincaid, J. P., Lance, S., & Hodgson, T. (1976). Spontaneous use of mnemonic and grade point average. *The Journal of Psychology, 92,* 117 - 122.

[12] O'Hara, R., et al. (2006). Long-term effects of mnemonic training in community-dwelling older adults. *Journal of Psychiatric Research, 41,* 585 – 590.

[13] Taguchi, K. (2006). Should the keyword method be introduced into tertiary foreign language classrooms? *Electronic Journal of Foreign Language Teaching, 3, (Suppl. 1),* 22 – 38.

[14] Atkinson, R. C., & Raugh, M. R., 1975). An

application of the mnemonic keyword method to the acquisition of a Russian vocabulary. *Journal of Experimental Psychology: Human learning and memory, 104,* 126 – 133.

[15] Nation, I.S. P. (2001). *Learning vocabulary in another language.* Cambridge, UK: Cambridge University Press.

[16] Atkinson, R. C., & Raugh, M. R., 1975). An application of the mnemonic keyword method to the acquisition of a Russian vocabulary. *Journal of Experimental Psychology: Human learning and memory, 104,* 126 – 133.

[17] Carney, R. N., & Levin, J. R. (2003). Promoting higher-order learning benefits by building lower-order mnemonic connections. *Applied Cognitive Psychology, 17,* 563 - 575. (p. 573 - 574).

[18] Carney, R. N., & Levin, J. R. (2003). Promoting higher-order learning benefits by building lower-order mnemonic connections. *Applied Cognitive Psychology, 17,* 563 - 575. (p. 572).

[19] Goldberg, S. (2011). *Clinical anatomy made ridiculously simple.* Miami, FL : MedMaster.

[20] Evans, R. L. (2007). *Every good boy deserves fudge.* New York: Perigee.

[21] Parkinson, J. (2008). *i before e (except after c).* Pleasantville, NY: Reader's Digest Association.

[22] Mirkin, G. & Rich, D. (1995). *Fat free, flavor full: Dr. Gabe Mirkin's guide to losing weight and living*

longer. New York: Hachette.

[23] Chowdhury, N. R. (2006). *Memory techniques for science students.* New Dehli: Fusion Books.

[24] Klaeser, B. M. (1977). *Reading improvement: a complete course for increasing speed and comprehension.* Chicago: Nelson-Hall.

[25] Young, C. V. (1971). *The magic of a mighty memory.* West Nyak, NY: Parker Publishing Company

[26] Evans, R. L. (2007). *Every good boy deserves fudge.* New York: Perigee.

[27] Bellezza, F. S. (1982). *Improve your memory skills.* Englewood Cliffs, NJ: Prentice Hall.

[28] Bellezza, F. S. (1982). *Improve your memory skills.* Englewood Cliffs, NJ: Prentice Hall.

[29] Borgman, D. A. (1965). *Language on vacation: An olio of orthographical oddities.* New York: Charles Scribner's Sons.

[30] Cukier, M. (1999). The final exam: Pi mnemonics. *Math Horizons, 6,* (4).

[31] Cleveland, W., & Alvarez, M. (1992). *Yo, Millard Filmore!: (And all those other Presidents you don't know).* Woodbury, CT: Fundamentals.

[32] Luria, A. R. (1968). The mind of a mnemonist: A little book about a vast memory. Cambridge, MA: Harvard University Press. (p. 49).

[33] Bellezza, F. S. (1981). Mnemonic devices: Classification, characteristics, and criteria. *Review of Educational Research, 51,* 247 - 275.

[34] Sambrook, J. (1889). *Phonographic systems of*

mnemonics: *Summary of class tuition*. Lincoln, UK: Akrill, Ruddick, & Keyworth.

[35] Scruggs, T. E., Mastropieri, M. A. & Levin, J. R. (1986). Can children effectively reuse the same mnemonic peg words? *Educational Technology Research and Development, 34,* 83 - 88.

[36] Buzan, T. (1991). *Use your perfect memory*. New York: Plume.

[37] Young, M. N. & Gibson, W. B. (1962). *How to develop an exceptional memory*. North Hollywood, CA: Melvin Powers - Wilshire Book Company.

[38] Fuller, H. H. (1898). *The art of memory: Being a comprehensive and practical system of memory culture*. St. Paul, MN: National Publishing Company.

[39] Maguire, E. A., Valentine, E. R., Wilding, J. M. & Kapur, N. (2003). Routes to remembering: The brains behind superior memory. *Nature Neuroscience, 6,* 90 - 95.

[40] Sherry, D. F., Jacobs, L. F., & Gaulin, S. J. (1992). Spatial memory and adaptive specialization of the hippocampus. Trends in neurosciences, 15(8), 298-303

[41] Shamburger, M. I., & Lachmann, V. R. (1946). Southey and" The Three Bears. The Journal of American Folklore, 59, 400-403.

[42] Foer, J., (2011). *Moonwalking with Einstein, The art and science of remembering everything*. New York:

The Penguin Press. (p. 44).

[43] Hale-Evans, R., & Hale-Evans, M. (2011). *Mindhacker*. Indianapolis, IN: Wiley Publishing.

[44] Norman, D. A. (1969). *Memory and attention: An introduction to human information processing*. New York: John Wiley & Sons.

[45] Baddeley, A., Eysenck, M. W., & Anderson, M. C. (2010). *Memory*. New York: Psychology Press.

[46] O'Brien, D. (2000). *Learn to remember: Practical techniques and exercises to improve your memory*. San Francisco; Chronicle Books.

[47] Middleton, A. E. (1888). *Memory systems: New and old*. New York: G. S. Fellows & Company.

[48] O'Brien, D. (2000). *Learn to remember: Practical techniques and exercises to improve your memory*. San Francisco; Chronicle Books. (p. 108).

[49] Buzan, T. (2004). *Master your memory*. London: BBC.

[50] Hulstijn, J. H. (1997). Mnemonic methods in foreign language vocabulary learning: Theoretical considerations and pedagogical implications. In J. Coady & T. Huckin (Eds.). *Second language vocabulary acquisition: A rationale for pedagogy*. (pp. 203 - 224). Cambridge, UK: Cambridge University Press.

[51] Vernon, D. V. (2009). *Human potential: Exploring techniques used to enhance human performance*. London: Routledge.

[52] Foer, J., (2011). *Moonwalking with Einstein, The art and science of remembering everything.* New York: The Penguin Press. (p. 267).

Chapter 8

Ebbinghaus and The Forgetting Curve

It's surprising it didn't drive him mad. Every day for months on end German Psychologist Hermann Ebbinghaus would learn and recite long lists of meaningless syllables. Whatever the tedium of these exercises, it was worth trouble. From these experiments, conducted in the 1880s, Ebbinghaus forged the modern science of memory.

Ebbinghaus was the first psychologist to perform rigorous memory experiments. After receiving his Ph.D. in 1873 Ebbinghaus spent two years teaching in England, where he came in contact with the associational psychology promoted by British philosophers. Also, while in England he came across a copy of the *Elements of Psychophysics* by Gustav Fechner, an early advocate of experimental psychology.

The great philosopher Immanuel Kant claimed that it was impossible to measure the mind. Fechner's work was a direct assault on this pessimistic view. He was able to find law like relationships in the way people responded to stimuli.[1] Ebbinghaus was deeply impressed with Fechner's arguments and felt that he might be able move the study of learning from philosophical speculation to verifiable research. He used himself as a subject and many of his early conclusions have been supported by subsequent research.

Ebbinghaus noted that the study of memory presented a central difficulty. If memory is affected by the degree of association, how could you control for past associations? Previous exposure might contaminate experimental results. If asked to memorize a line of poetry, previous exposure, even unremembered exposure, might affect your current ability to commit the line to memory. To solve this problem Ebbinghaus hit upon the use of three letter nonsense syllables, often called trigrams. Each trigram consisted of two consonants separated by a vowel, such as MIB or LAJ.

In a typical experiment, Ebbinghaus would create a deck of thirteen cards with a single trigram on each card. He placed a blank card on the top of the deck.

On the first trial he would go through the deck turning over each card, trying to learn the cards in order. After the first trial the he would turn to the deck over and start again, but this time when he looked at the blank card on the top he would try to name the following card. He would then turn over the blank card and see if he was correct. Looking at the first trigram card he would try to guess the name of the second trigram card and so on through the deck. This is called the method of serial anticipation, because he had to recall, that is anticipate, the next card from looking at the card that preceded it.

Even though Ebbinghaus was working with nonsense syllables the method of serial anticipation, essentially a type of list learning, did resemble many important memory tasks. For example, learning the alphabet, the correct spelling of a word, or the lines of a poem, requires us to recall information in a particular order where each item is a cue for the next one.[2]

When Ebbinghaus could work through the deck without error twice he considered the deck learned and recorded the total time it had taken him to learn the deck.

After a deck was learned he would wait some amount of time, sometimes minutes, sometimes days, and test himself again. Typically he would make some mistakes and he would work through the deck a number of times to in order to relearn it. As with initial learning he considered the deck relearned if he could he could work through it twice without error.

Not surprisingly it took less time to relearn the deck. The amount of time it took to learn the deck originally minus the time it took to relearn he called the "savings," a measure of how much work had been saved in relearning the deck over initial learning. Dividing the savings by the amount of time it first took to learn the deck allowed him to represent the information saved in memory as a decimal fraction.[3]

By repeating this experiment many times with many different list over many different time intervals, Ebbinghaus made several important discoveries that bear on our goal of memory improvement. Perhaps, the most important was a pattern that emerged over his many experiments, a relationship between initial learning, time, and forgetting that we have come to call the forgetting curve. The forgetting curve is essentially the opposite of the learning curve;[4] the downward slope of the curve shows us how much information is lost over time. Studying this curve will lead us to understand those factors that increase resistance to forgetting.

The Forgetting Curve

"Speaking generally, whatever may be the nature of the traces left in our minds by our experiences, those traces gradually fade, and the curve of remembering has but one tendency — a downward tendency." — Philip Ballard[5]

The forgetting curve is a simple graph of the relationship between retention and time. The horizontal x-axis represents time while the y-axis represents the amount of material retained. Ebbinghaus found that he typically forgot one-third of the material in the first 20 minutes. After this initial sharp drop, forgetting would become slower; it took nine additional hours to forget the next third of the material. Between 9 and 24 hours forgetting continued but at an even slower rate.[6]

Psychologist Harry Bahrick of Ohio Wesleyan University, has attempted to investigate the forgetting curve over the course of the life span. In one experiment he tested the ability of high school alumni to recognize their classmates, by name or from yearbook photos, 25 years after graduation. In this case, he found that there was little forgetting, and the classic forgetting curve did not seem to apply. However, when he tested college professors for memory of students names and faces he found that forgetting began almost immediately after the end of the semester. By eight years after the end of the semester, the instructors had almost no ability to recognize their former students. Bahrick explained the differences in performance in terms of initial learning. High school classmates had four years of interaction in many situations with their classmates, while the professors were only exposed to their students in the classroom a few times a week for a ten week quarter.[7]

Students had better memory of their classmates because of two factors that changed the slope of the forgetting curve in a more favorable direction, over-learning and distributed practice. Over-learning is when we continue to study information even after we reach mastery. Distributed practice is when the rehearsal of learned information is spread out over many sessions rather than condensed into one or a few sessions. [8] Unlike the professors, whose interaction with the students was very limited in time, the constant interactions between the students themselves acted as a both over-learning and distributed practice.

In a later study, Bahrick looked at how much people retained from taking Spanish language classes years after leaving school. The pattern of forgetting followed Ebbinghaus's curve and memory declined exponentially for the first three to six years. After that the retention of the remaining information remained stable for decades. Much of the information was still retained at 50 years after completing Spanish classes. Since most graduates did not practice or review during these long intervals, individual differences in performance were mostly the result of different levels of initial training.

One important consequence of the Bahrick study

is that is shows that academic training does contribute to the long term knowledge base of students. Graduates often claim they cannot remember anything they learned in school, but this is a mis-perception. While a significant amount of information is lost, a sizable portion of the information taught in school does take a place in our long term memory. Bahrick wrote of a "permastore"[9] that held academic information over a lifetime. Educators need to find ways to increase the amount of information in this permastore.

The science of memory improvement is the study of the factors that alter the curve of forgetting. For example, one early study compared the forgetting curves for meaningless trigrams and poetry. Poetry, material with meaning, was better remembered than the meaningless syllables.[10] Thus, different types of material will have different curves. In general, the curve for meaningless material will fall sharply. While the curve for meaningful material will have a slower descent.

Why We Forget

We cannot remember everything. Or at least most of us can't. As I have noted, there have been a handful of people, such as Solomon Shereshevsky or Kim Peek, with remarkable, seemingly total, recall. However, this level of memory is beyond the reach of most of us and forgetting seems to be a feature of the average brain. Yet it is possible to substantially improve the memory performance of our average brains. In order to do this though we must have a deeper understanding of forgetting.

The Romans believed that reading tombstone epitaphs caused forgetting, but this no longer seems a plausible explanation.[11] There are several hypotheses to explain why we forget.

One fact worth noting is that the mind and its memory systems evolved for a world in which we no longer live. Most of us tend to be good at remembering place and spatial information, skills that would have been valuable for our hunter gatherer ancestors. For example, it may surprise you that we have superior memory for animal tracks. One study reported that contemporary college students did better on memory tests for animal tracks than for other categories of objects. The other categories were armored vehicles, sea shells, unusual kitchen utensils, trees. While the students had the best memory for kitchen utensils, they also did quite well at animal tracks, significantly better than the other groups of objects. Even though they had little experience with and professed little interest in animal tracks, they still had better memory for them. This research suggests that we have a biological predisposition to learn certain types of information, a product of selective forces that shaped the brain of our ancestors.[12]

Our memory system is less well equipped for the culturally created symbolic environment that we now inhabit. Our brains did not evolve to remember ATM pin numbers or the axioms of geometry. However, if can understand the underlying principals of forgetting and remembering we can develop techniques that allow us to cope better with the memory demands of the modern world.

Ebbinghaus showed that memory is a function of the strength of the initial memory and the passage of time. This relationship defines the forgetting curve. Initial memory strength may account for the phenomenon of flashbulb memory, where we vividly remember some shocking or life changing events such as the attack on September 11th. Flashbulb memories can be important historical events or they can be significant personal experiences. Improved memory for single occurrence events seems to violate the idea that repetition is necessary for memory. Thus, this phenomenon requires special explanation, and it could be that the initial intensity of these memories start the forgetting curve at a higher place and, thus, the forgetting curve has further to fall. However, there is controversy over both the accuracy of Flashbulb memories and their cause. It is possible that we remember these events simply because we repeat, rehearse, and discuss them frequently.[13]

While flashbulb memories may or may not be examples of initial memory strength, studies of long term memories have consistently shown that the stronger an earlier memory, the longer it is retained. For instance, you will retain more information for a longer time from a class where your grade was A than one where your grade was C.

The passage of time is the second factor defining the forgetting curve. If you are asked about a newspaper article shortly after reading it, your recall is likely to be good, if you are asked a week later you are unlikely to be able to recall much.[14] In general more recent information is more accessible than older information, a phenomenon known as the long term recency effect.[15]

One important feature of the forgetting curve is that the curve falls in a predictable fashion. It falls steeply at first and then the falls less sharply. Thus, most forgetting occurs shortly after learning. The slope of the curve is similar regardless of the amount learned. This means that students will forget at about the same rate even if they learn at a different rates.[16] Of course, the student who learns more will retain more information, but in the absence of mnemonic strategies the memory curves will follow the same downward pattern.

There is no doubt that there is a difference in how fast we learn. For example, some students learn course material rapidly with very little review, while other students will learn the same material much more slowly. However, even if two different students take different amounts of time to learn the same information, once learned they will forget at about the same rates. [17] Educators make a distinction between aptitude and achievement. Aptitude refers to some potentiality that inheres in the individual and an aptitude test tries to measure that potential. Speed of learning might be considered an aptitude. Achievement, on the other hand, is the actual mastery of material. In the school context, achievement refers to whether you mastered the material that was taught. It is possible that a student with a faster learning speed may not bother to study the material. The student with the slower learning speed may outperform the faster student through hard work. An aptitude for fast learning, while a great advantage, is of no value if it is not applied. Moreover, if upon learning the material the slower learner applies some of the memory principles described in this book much more of that information can be retained. As we will see, there are techniques that can alter the slope of the forgetting curve.

The Nature of Forgetting — Decay and Interference

Psychologists makes a distinction between information being lost *from* memory and information being lost *in* memory. Information is lost from memory when the memory trace decays or is destroyed. When information is lost in memory, the memory trace still exists but the retrieval process fails. We might use the library as an analogy. You cannot access an old book if it has decayed into dust. This is an issue for librarians, books printed on acid based paper do decay rapidly. On the other hand, the library may posses the book but have mis-shelved it.[18] I have occasionally discovered books at my university library where the Library Congress number on the book's spine did not match the number entered into the catalog. In these cases, the book may be in the library's collection, but irretrievable.

One early explanation for forgetting was proposed by the psychologist Edward Thorndike, the Law of Disuse.[19] Now generally called the decay theory, the idea here is that memories (or the associations between memories) have a tendency to weaken and to decay over time.[20]

But while decay seems intuitive, many psychologists have questioned if it is the correct explanation for forgetting. If the decay theory is true then there must be some time dependent process in the nervous system that cause memories to weaken. Behaviorally oriented psychologists have been reluctant to accept the existence of internal factors as an explanation for memory performance. They have preferred to look for environmental causes for forgetting.[21] While this approach is unnecessarily limiting, it did lead to a powerful alternative explanation for forgetting, interference.

The interference theory was proposed in 1932 by John Alexander McGeoch. The idea here is that information is not forgotten as much as lost due to interference between associations.[22] The associations formed by a new memory might either block or compete with existing associations. When we learn something, we may make an association between a single retrieval cue and a memory. If that cue also becomes associated with a different memory, then the two memories become in competition with each other. Information is not destroyed but becomes unavailable through a process of interference, memories in competition with each other. As more memories become associated with a single cue increases the probability of recalling the desired information decreases, this is called cue-overload.[23]

At the beginning of this book, I mentioned my difficulty remembering the name of singer Willie Nelson and suggested that it might be caused by an interfering memory. In this case, the interfering memory is another person, Woody Starr, who also has long hair and wears a cowboy hat. Woody and I have talked about Willie and their first names start with the same letter. Many of the cues that should call up Willie's names also call up Woody's. The information is still in my memory, but interference makes it difficult to find it.

Evidence for interference can be found in the work of Ebbinghaus, a highly original and intelligent scientist. Because he used himself as a subject and published his results it is possible to compare his performance with participants in subsequent similar experiments. The results are surprising, while these studies have confirmed the existence of the forgetting curve, most participants show less forgetting than Ebbinghaus. One possible explanation for his inferior performance is that he used himself as a subject in repeated experiments. In most other experiments the participants are tested only once or a few times. Ebbinghaus tested himself repeatedly for many years and psychologist have speculated that the previously learned material interfered with his attempts to learn new lists of nonsense syllables.[24]

Interference provides an another explanation for why we forget where we parked the car. The idea here is that interference is stronger when memories are similar. You might recall in the movie *Twelve Angry Men*, Juror Eight, played by Henry Fonda, questions Juror Four, E. G. Marshall, about his memory. As the questions reach further back in time Juror Eight's memory for his mundane daily activity becomes less certain. If we do something unusual or only once we might form only one memory trace strongly linked a specific cue. On the other hand, when we do something similar each new memory trace becomes a competitor for the same cue. Thus, we might be likely to remember where we parked our car at our first visit to a new shopping center, and less likely when we park at the grocery store we visit every week. We've parked in many different spaces at the grocery store, and all those memories are in competition. This implies that routine behaviors produce more interference and are likely to be less memorable.[25]

Interference plays a role in some tip of the tongue forgetting. When we fail to retrieve the information we want, we often feel blocked by some similar piece of information.[26] This was the case when I tried to remember Willie Nelson's name but could only come up with Woody's.

We can also see the effect of interference in foreign language learning. When we first learn a word in a foreign language we usually make an association between the new word and its translation in our native tongue. For example, the Japanese word for dog is *inu*. Upon learning this fact, we forge a single association between *inu* and dog. However, we already have many associations with the word dog: the dog we had as a child, the names of the many dog breeds, the neighbor's dog who barks all night, and so on. Thus, we have many strong associations competing with the single association to the word in Japanese.[27]

Surprisingly, a second language may be harder to learn when its sounds are similar to the sounds of the native language. A language with a dramatically different pattern of pronunciation may provide less interference[28]

Interference has also been proposed as an explanation for flashbulb memories, where we seem to have particularity vivid memories of highly unusual events. Unusual events by their very nature are dissimilar to other memories and, thus, are subject to less interference.

Interference could also explain why certain learning tasks are difficult. Memorizing basic math facts means learning many items that are highly similar to each other. A math fact taught in elementary school consists of two number separated by an operator symbol (+, -, x, or /). This degree of similarity between items increases the chance of interference and makes memory more difficult.[29]

There is also some evidence that auditory memories are more susceptible to interference than visual images, and this might explain why imagery is so effective as a memory aid.[30]

Errors in initial learning can also be a source of interference. If we first spell a word incorrectly, that incorrect spelling may cause us problems. The memory of the incorrect spelling does not go away, rather, it is stored in memory and interferes with the memory of the correct spelling. Some educators have advocated the use of invented spelling and not correcting children when they make errors such as writing backwards.[31] This approach may have the unintended consequence of creating greater interference.[32] This makes a compelling case for the use of errorless learning of basic skills. In errorless learning, the process of learning is broken down into small incremental steps so that errors are rarely made.[33]

Errorless learning is different from trial and error learning. In trial and error learning we must distinguish between a correct response and an incorrect response. We learn which response is correct because it is reinforced in some way. We learn which response is incorrect because it is either has no consequence or has a corrective or punitive consequence.[34]

While we learn many things through trial and error learning, there is a danger that if we initially make the incorrect response, it will interfere with our memory of the correct response. For example, a student who answers a question incorrectly on an exam might then tend to remember the wrong answer. In errorless learning the teacher structures instruction to minimize the chances of an incorrect response.

However, errorless learning is a goal that is not always achieved. While it is possible to reduce the number of errors that a student makes it not possible to eliminate them. We can still reduce the effect of error interference through the use of immediate feedback. Intimidate feedback means presenting the correct answer before the next question is asked, or the next problem is begun. The effect of immediacy is important. It is not immediate feedback to provide the answers after the student has completed the worksheet. Immediate feedback comes before the student begins the next problem.[35] The reduction of error interference through immediate feedback is a technique that could be more widely used in classrooms at all levels of education. An example of one technique is immediate feedback grading, as developed by Beth and Mike Epstein, which allows students to see if their answers are correct immediately after responding. There is good evidence for the effectiveness of this technique and it is unfortunate that is not well known by educators.[36]

The observation that sleep seemed to improve memory was taken as being evidence that interference was the driving force in forgetting. People will have better memory for a list of nonsense words if, after studying them, they sleep than if they stay awake for the same amount of time. Many psychologists concluded that memory improves with sleep because it shuts out interfering information.[37] However, there are other plausible explanations. Indeed, there is evidence that sleep directly strengthens memory traces.[38]

It is very difficult to decide between the interference and the decay theory. This is because failure to remember proves only that the memory is inaccessible at that time, not that decay has occurred. Once while visiting a comic book convention with my son, I saw a comic book for sale that I had read as a child. If you had asked me about it in advance, I would not have been able to remember it. At that point, I might have concluded that my memory had decayed to nothing. But when I saw the cover I immediately remembered having read it and some details of the plot. Seeing the cover opened up memories that were previously inaccessible, lost in memory but not from memory.[39] To add insult to injury, the comic book now had a price tag that was considerably higher than the 12 cents I had paid as a kid.

Is there an experiment that could help us decide between the interference and the decay explanation of forgetting? For the case of working term memory,

Psychologists Nancy Waugh and Donald Norman devised what they called the probe digit experiment to try to settle the issue. In this experiment, a person is presented with a series of 15 digits displayed one at a time. At the end of the series, the participant is shown a number that appeared only once on the list (the probe digit) and asked to name the digit that followed immediately after the probe digit.

For example, the digits 6 5 6 3 5 4 9 7 8 7 2 5 4 1 6 might be read to the participant one at a time. At the end of the sequence, the participant would be asked to name the digit that occurred after 9, a probe digit that occurred only once in the list. The correct answer would be 7. Since the probe digit occurs only once in the list, there could only be one correct answer.

Both the interference and the decay hypothesis predict better memory for digits that appeared later in the list. In the case of interference, it was because there would be more interference for digits that appeared early in the list. On the other hand since more time had elapsed since the first digits had been presented there would be more time for the information to decay. However, Waugh and Norman believed that they could distinguish between decay and interference by presenting the list at different speeds. In the fast condition, digits were presented at the rate of four per second. In the slow condition the digits were presented one per second. If the decay contributed to forgetting then memory for earlier digits would be better in the fast condition since the time between first seeing digit and recall would be shorter. There would be less time for forgetting. If interference was the cause of forgetting then only the position of a digit on the list should affect recall.[40]

While the experimental procedure was straightforward, the interpretation of the results was not. A typical textbook synopsis of Waugh's and Norman's findings tells us "they found that time intervals had no effect; performance was much better predicted by number of intervening digits."[41] Notice, however, that the sentence is ambiguous, almost self contradictory. In the first phrase it is claimed that the different time interval had no effect. However, the second phrase acknowledges the time interval did have an effect, albeit a weak one. While the Waugh and Norman study had been taken as evidence against the decay hypothesis, a reanalysis of the data shows that when the presentation rate was faster there was an improvement in memory for digits earlier on the list. This decay effect was in addition to a substantial interference effect.

Thus, our best evidence is that *both* decay and interference contribute to forgetting in working memory. Indeed, if interference is the only factor that causes forgetting then interference would, over time, make it impossible to remember anything. Every new fact learned becomes a source of interference and eventually the system would become swamped with interfering associations. There must then be some other forgetting process that thins out the competing memory traces and decay seems the most reasonable explanation.[42]

One of the main criticisms of the decay theory has been the observation that time is not itself a cause. Iron rusts over time but time is not the cause of rust, rather the cause of rust is oxidation.[43] But this argument is flawed. Of course, a claim that a process is time dependent is inadequate without the discovery of an underlying mechanism. However, it does not make the fact of time dependency false.

Indeed, we now can find examples of underlying mechanisms of memory decay. For example, there is considerable evidence that as we age there are physical changes in the brain, including declines in synaptic connectivity and the efficacy of the brain's neurotransmitters, that provide a plausible biological explanation for age related memory decay.[44] In addition, research examining the underlying neurobiology of memory has found plausible examples of structural decay tied to memory loss. Research on sea snail neurons has found synaptic changes associated with the acquisition of a new memory and the decay of those changes associated with the loss of that memory.[45]

Memories may differ in their susceptibility to decay. This vulnerability to decay is called the fragility of a memory. The more fragile a memory the more likely it is to decay. Memories tend to become less fragile overtime so in general newer memories are the most fragile, the most likely to decay and to be forgotten. Jost's Law is the observation that if two memories are of equal strength, the older memory will be retained longer. This can be observed in many amnesic patients who are able to recover older memories but not more recent ones.[46]

Fragility can also be described in terms of its inverse, consolidation. Hebb had suggested that memories begin as patterns of brain cell activity.[47]

These patterns, since they do not involve structural changes to the brain, are inherently fragile. Over the learning process, those memories that are reinforced are consolidated into structural changes in the brain.[48]

We have already discussed how damage to the hippocampus can lead to a permanent inability to consolidate new long term memories. Other factors, such as, concussion and electro-convulsive therapy, can also disrupt consolidation. It has long been known that people who suffer head trauma often do not remember the events that occurred immediately prior to the injury. [49] Physician Martin Luther Holbrook gives several examples of this in his 1886 book, *How to Strengthen the Memory*. Benjamin Franklin accidentally shocked himself while trying to test the effects of electricity on a turkey. He reported that it "took him some minutes to recollect his thoughts."[50]

Electro-convulsive therapy is a procedure used to treat individuals with severe depression that cannot be treated with drugs or cognitive-behavioral therapy. Under anesthesia electrodes are placed on patients head and an electric current is passed through the brain. This technique is extremely effective in reducing the symptoms of depression. However, patients often experience memory problems after the treatment. Electro-convulsive therapy interferes with the consolidation of memories and provides an opportunity to study the process. One clever study looked at patients' memory for television shows and found that the electro-convulsive therapy disrupted memories that occurred one to two years before treatment, but not prior to that.[51]

Thus, the consolidation of information into long term memory is a process that occurs over several years. We need the hippocampus to form and maintain long term memories, but after a period of about three years the information consolidates into long term memory and the hippocampus is no longer necessary to access it.[52]

Retrieval Failure

We have all experienced retrieval failure in tip of the tongue states, where we could not recall a name, but were able to remember it at some later time. We can show that retrieval failure is real by comparing recall to recognition memory. In a typical experiment, volunteers were shown 100 words five times and asked to recall and many as possible. On average the volunteers could only come up with 37 words. However, when asked to identify the 100 words from a list that included 100 words not presented, on average they were able to identify 96 correctly.[53] Clearly, the information was stored in memory, otherwise they would not have been able to distinguish between the two sets of words.

Tip of the tongue states allow us to study how memory works. Normally the process of recall is seamless; we need a word and we draw it out of our long term memory store in a tiny fraction of a second. In the tip of the tongue situation this process breaks down. We look for the word but cannot find it. Tip of the tongue forgetting is often associated with the feeling that one knows the concept but not the specific word. Thus, there appears to be two different entities in our memory: first, an abstract conceptual representation (called the lemma) that included its meaning and its grammatical functional and, second, the phonetic, sound, representation of that concept (known as the lexeme). Thus, the tip of the tongue state is a kind of complex forgetting where we can recover the lemma but cannot associate it with the correct lexeme. This fact disproves a widely held belief that we cannot have concepts without words.[54]

The Repression Theory of Forgetting

Slips of the tongue are also a kind of forgetting. Here we recover the wrong word or put words in the wrong order. A classic example of this is the spoonerism. Named after the Oxford Don William Archibald Spooner, who exhibited this interesting verbal behavior. A spoonerism is where the first parts of words are accidentally exchanged, sometimes with humorous results. For example, instead of asking "is the dean busy?" one might say "is the bean dizzy?"[55]

Amusing stories of spoonerisms raises the question, do slips of the tongue represent failed attempts to repress embarrassing thoughts? This notion is associated with Freud's theory of repression. Freud believed that we unconsciously repress embarrassing or anxiety provoking memories. His theory of repression is, in fact, a theory of forgetting.

In 1976 psychologist Alan Baddeley reviewed evidence for repression forgetting and did find some evidence in favor of this hypothesis. For example, there is a psychiatric state called "psychogenic fugue."[56] Fugue is a kind of amnesia often induced by severe emotional trauma. It includes wandering, and loss of identity and autobiographical memories. Although there is evidence of some fugue states being caused by physical traumas most are induced by psychological trauma. Generally, physical trauma will induce anterograde amnesia, where an individual has trouble forming new long term memories. In retrogrades amnesias, such as fugue, a person is unable to access existing long term memories. These tend to have a psychological cause.[57]

This suggests, as Freud believed, that at least some forms of forgetting are emotional in origin. Jung's word association experiments have some bearing on this issue. In an association test a person is given a word and is then asked to say the first word that comes to mind. Jung measured how long it took to produce an answer and discovered that emotionally charged words had longer delays. This implies that recovery from memory might be influenced by emotional factors.

We also know that the hedonic content of information affects memory. Hedonic means related to pleasure. Most people are more likely to remember pleasant information than unpleasant information. This does seem to support Freud's notion of repression, suggesting that we might repress unpleasant memories. However, the difference is small and we are, also, more likely to remember information both pleasant and unpleasant more than neutral information. In addition, more pessimistic people reverse the usual pattern and have better memory for unpleasant information.[58]

At least some of forgetting associated with traumatic events may be caused by sleep disruption rather than repression. It has long been known that there is an association between traumatic events, amnesia, and sleep disorders. Instead of repression, it is possible that problems with sleep, such as insomnia after a traumatic event are a cause of memory disruption.[59]

At the end of his review of the repression theory, Baddeley concluded that "while it seems likely that repression does occasionally occur in everyday life, it can surly not account for more than a minute fraction of the vast amount of information we process and forget every day."[60]

Poincare's Forgetting Hypothesis.

One final idea about forgetting that is worthy of consideration is Poincare's forgetting hypothesis. Henri Poincare, a brilliant mathematician and physicist, whose work anticipated Einstein's theory of relativity, noticed that he often made important discoveries after he forgot about a problem. He described situations where after working on a problem he would put aside and forget about it. Later the solution would come to him in a flash of insight at an unexpected time. This suggests that there is some kind of unconscious information processing occurs with information in long term memory under the guise of forgetting.

One review of accounts of scientific creativity found a similar pattern to the one described by Poincare. There was first a period of intense work on the problem, a preparation stage, where the individual engages in intense mental effort to solve a problem. After a while, the person gives up trying to solve the problem. But in the unconscious memory the problem is still being processed. Sometimes a solution pops out in an eureka moment.[61]

Here unconscious memory acts as a kind of incubator. Perhaps, when we try to solve difficult problems in our conscious mind we are too often plagued by interference that prevents us from exploring new approaches to the problem. According to this view while interference is the source of some kinds of forgetting, in some cases we experience a temporary forgetting that may suppress interference.

---

[1] Garrett, H. E. (1951). *Great experiments in psychology.* New York: Appleton-Crofts.

[2] Bower, G. H. (2000) A brief history of memory research. In E. Tulving & F. I. M. Craik (Eds.). *The Oxford handbook of memory* (pp. 3- 32). Oxford: Oxford University Press.

[3] Ebbinghaus, H. (1913/1964). *Memory: A contribution to experimental psychology.* (Trans. H. A. Ruger & C. E. Bussenius). New York: Dover Publications.

[4] Radvansky, G. A. (2011). *Human memory.* Boston; Allyn & Bacon.

[5] Ballard, P. B. (1913). *Obliviscence and Reminiscence.* Cambridge, UK: Cambridge University Press. (p. 1)

[6] Bean, C. H. (1912). *The curve of forgetting.* New York: New Era.

[7] Bahrick, H. P. (1984). Semantic memory content in permastore: Fifty years of memory for Spanish Learned in School. *Journal of Experimental Psychology: General, 113,* 1 - 29

[8] Radvansky, G. A. (2011). *Human memory.* Boston; Allyn & Bacon.

[9] Bahrick, H. P. (1984). Semantic memory content in permastore: Fifty years of memory for Spanish Learned in School. *Journal of Experimental Psychology: General, 113,* 1 - 29. (p. 1).

[10] Bean, C. H. (1912). *The curve of forgetting.* New York: New Era.

[11] Shenk, D. (2003). *The forgetting: Alzheimer's: Portrait of an epidemic.* New York: Anchor Books.

[12] Sharps, M. J., Villegas, A., Nunes, M. A., & Barber, T. L. (2002). Memory for Animal Tracks: A Possible Cognitive Artifact of Human Evolution. *Journal Of Psychology, 136,* 469 - 492.

[13] Cohen, G. (1989). *Memory in the real world.* Hove, UK: Lawrence Erlbaum Associates

[14] Parkin, A. J. (1990). *Memory and amnesia: An introduction.* Cambridge, MA: Basil Blackwell.

[15] Baddeley, A., Eysenck, M. W., & Anderson, M. C. (2010). *Memory.* New York: Psychology Press.

[16] Wickelgren, W. A. (1977). *Learning and memory.* Englewood Cliffs, NJ: Prentice-Hall Inc.

[17] Thompson, R. F., & Madigan, S. A. (2005). *Memory: The key to consciousness. Washington*, D.C.: Joseph Henry Press.

[18] Baddeley, A. D. (1976). *The psychology of memory.* New York: Basic Books.

[19] Thorndike, E. L. (1913). *Educational Psychology: Volume II; The original nature of man.* New York: Teachers College, Columbia University.

[20] Parkin, A. J. (1990). *Memory and amnesia: An introduction.* Cambridge, MA: Basil Blackwell.

[21] Lutz, J. (2005). *Learning and memory.* Long Grove, IL: Waveland Press.

[22] McGeoch, J. A., (1932). Forgetting and the Law of Disuse. *Psychology Review, 39,* pp. 352-370.

[23] Baddeley, A., Eysenck, M. W., & Anderson, M. C. (2010). *Memory.* New York: Psychology Press.

[24] Lutz, J. (2005). *Learning and memory.* Long Grove, IL: Waveland Press.

[25] Baddeley, A., Eysenck, M. W., & Anderson, M. C. (2010). *Memory.* New York: Psychology Press.

[26] Weinland, J. D. (1957). *How to improve your memory.* New York: Barnes and Noble, Inc.

[27] Nation, I.S. P. (2001). *Learning vocabulary in another language.* Cambridge, UK: Cambridge University Press.

[28] Nation, I.S. P. (2001). *Learning vocabulary in another language.* Cambridge, UK: Cambridge University Press.

[29] Wickelgren, W. A. (1977). *Learning and memory.* Englewood Cliffs, NJ: Prentice-Hall Inc.

[30] Wickelgren, W. A. (1977). *Learning and memory.* Englewood Cliffs, NJ: Prentice-Hall Inc.

[31] Routman, R. (1991). *Invitations: Changing as teachers and learners K - 12.* Portsmouth, NH: Heinemann

[32] Wickelgren, W. A. (1977). *Learning and memory.* Englewood Cliffs, NJ: Prentice-Hall Inc.

[33] Vargas, J. S. (2009). *Behavior analysis for effective teaching.* New York: Routledge.

[34] Mueller, M. M., Palkovic, C. M., & Maynard, C. S. (2007). Errorless learning: Review and practical application for teaching children with pervasive developmental delay. *Psychology in the Schools, 44,* 691 - 700.

[35] Vargas, J. S. (2009). *Behavior analysis for effective teaching.* New York: Routledge.

[36] Epstein, M. L., Lazarus, A. D., Calvano, T. B., Matthews, K. A., Hendel, R. A., Epstein, B. B., & Brosvic, G. M. (2010). Immediate feedback assessment technique promotes learning and corrects inaccurate first responses. The Psychological Record, 52(2), 5.

[37] Stern, L. (1985). *The structures and strategies of human memory.* Homewood, IL: The Dorsey Press.

[38] Baddeley, A., Eysenck, M. W., & Anderson, M. C. (2010). *Memory.* New York: Psychology Press.

[39] Baddeley, A., Eysenck, M. W., & Anderson, M. C. (2010). *Memory*. New York: Psychology Press.

[40] Waugh, N. C. & Norman, D. A., (1965). Primary memory. *Psychological Review, 72*, 89 -104.

[41] Lutz, J. (2005). *Learning and memory*. Long Grove, IL: Waveland Press. (p. 260).

[42] Altmann, E. M., & Schunn, C. D. (2002). Integrating decay and interference: A new look at an old interaction. *Proceedings of the 24th annual meeting of the Cognitive Science Society* (pp. 65–70). Hillsdale, NJ: Erlbaum.

[43] McGeoch, J. A., (1932). Forgetting and the Law of Disuse. *Psychology Review, 39*, pp. 352-370.

[44] Fuster, J. M. (1999). *Memory in the cerebral cortex*. Cambridge, MA: MIT Press.

[45] Bailey,C. H., & Chen, M. (1989). Time course of structural changes identified sensory neuron synapses during long-term sensitization in *Aplysia*. *The Journal of Neuroscience, 9*, 1774 - 1780.

[46] Stern, L. (1985). *The structures and strategies of human memory*. Homewood, IL: The Dorsey Press.

[47] Hebb, D. O. (1949). *The organization of behavior: A neurophysical theory*. New York: John Wiley & Sons.

[48] Stern, L. (1985). *The structures and strategies of human memory*. Homewood, IL: The Dorsey Press.

[49] Holbrook, M. L. (1886). *How to strengthen the memory; Or, natural and scientific methods of*

never forgetting. New York: M. L. Holbrook & Company

[50] Franklin, B.(1809). *The Works of Benjamin Franklin* (vol. 3) Philadelphia: W. Colburn. (p. 135).

[51] Squire, L. R., & Cohen, N. (1979). Memory and amnesia: resistance to disruption develops for years after learning. Behavioral and neural biology, 25(1), 115-125.

[52] Winson, J. (1985). *Brain and psyche: The biology of the unconscious.* Garden City, NJ: Anchor Press.

[53] Mandler, G., Pearlstone, Z., & Koopman, H. S. (1969). Effects of organization and semantic similarity on recall and recognition. *Journal of Verbal Learning and Verbal Behavior, 8,* 410 - 423.

[54] Bucke, M. B. (2009). *Cosmic consciousness: A study in the evolution of the human mind.* Mineola, NY: Dover Publications.

[55] Hayter, W. (1977). *Spooner: A biography.* London: W. H. Allen

[56] Baddeley, A. D. (1976). *The psychology of memory.* New York: Basic Books.

[57] Parkin, A. J. (1990). *Memory and amnesia: An introduction.* Cambridge, MA: Basil Blackwell.

[58] Weinland, J. D. (1957). *How to improve your memory.* New York: Barnes and Noble, Inc.

[59] Van der Kloet, D. , et al. (2011). Fragmented sleep, fragmented mind: The role of sleep in dissociative symptoms. *Perspectives in Psychological Science, 7,*

159 - 175.

[60] Baddeley, A. D. (1976). *The psychology of memory.* New York: Basic Books. (p. 51).

[61] Hadamard, J. (1945). *An essay on the psychology of invention in the mathematical fields.* New York: Dover.

Chapter 9

Reversing the Forgetting Curve

In the last chapter, I described the forgetting curve, the discovery by Herman Ebbinghaus that forgetting occurs in a predictable pattern. From studying the forgetting curve, psychologists have identified four factors that affect retention. These factors are: 1) memory strength, 2) repetition, 3) the spacing effect, and 4) the testing effect. In this chapter, I will explain these factors and describe how you can use them to improve your memory.

Strength of Initial Memory

An important factor in remembering is the strength of the initial memory. When other factors are held constant, we forget at about the same rate. Yet even with similar rates of forgetting there will be differences in the amount of information remembered. This is because we start at different points on the forgetting curve. Remember that the height of the curve indicates how much we retain. If we start at a higher point than someone else, later we would still be at a higher point, assuming the rate of forgetting is the same. This has been verified in long term studies of memory for school material.[1] Years after leaving school, students who received As in class remember more than students who only received Cs.[2]

I have already noted the phenomenon of the flashbulb memory where we have better memory for emotionally intense or startling events.. To speak in the language of the forgetting curve, we would say that the intensity of the memory means a higher initial point on the curve. As we have seen in our discussion of mnemonics, an intense, bizarre, or unusual visual image is better remembered. An intense image creates a stronger initial memory.

Another way to manipulate the strength of an initial memory is overlearning. Ebbinghaus labeled a deck of nonsense syllables as learned when he could work through the stack of cards twice without error. In one set of experiments, he continued to study the list even after he had learned it. When he did this, he found he remembered more on subsequent trials. Overlearning means studying beyond the point of mastery. Students often make the mistake of ending study once they have mastered the material. If, instead, they continued to review the material, the more likely they would be to remember it.

Repetition

We all know from direct experience that repetition improves memory. When we memorized a poem or the Gettysburg address in school, we used rote repetition. The principle that repetition improves memory is well known by advertisers.[3] That is why we have to watch the same annoying commercials over and over again.

Why is our mind programmed to remember repeated information? Remembering events that occur with a frequency above some threshold must be adaptive. If we are likely to meet similar events in the future, we would do well to have profited from our experience. Studies of the brain have helped explain the underlying biology of repetition memory. When we study information over again we activate the same brain regions that we activated when we first learned that information. Put simply, repetition of previously stored information increases the strength of the memory trace.[4]

Repetition has two effects on the memory curve. First it brings the strength of memory back to its original level or higher. Second, it changes the slope of the forgetting curve towards greater retention.

Of course, repetition, often called rote memory, is much despised. It certainly can be boring. For some information, however, rote repetition may be necessary. For example, memorizing basic math facts. Fluency with basic math facts contributes to understanding higher level mathematics. Some math facts can be learned by the application of simple rules, such as the rule any number multiplied by zero is zero. However, many math facts do not lend themselves to that approach. If you want to learn that 7 x 8= 56, you will need to commit it to memory.

Fortunately, there are ways to make repetition less painful. Instead of cramming all the repetitions into a single mind numbing session we could spread those repetitions out over time and take advantage of the spacing effect.

Spacing Effect

The more time you spend learning something, the more you will remember. This observation, called the total time hypothesis, is not surprising. [5] What surprised many researchers was that memory also depended on how that practice was distributed.

During World War II, the military employed psychologist and educational innovator Fred Keller to improve the effectiveness of Morse code training. The demands of the war dramatically increased the need for Morse code operators and discovering an effective training regimen affected how quickly an operator could be put in the field. Code training was not an academic exercise, but something that had military consequences.[6]

Keller compared two groups of trainees, one trained for seven hours a day for five weeks and the other trained for four hours a day for eight weeks. Even though, the hours of study were almost the same, the group who practiced only four hours a day, distributed over a longer period, achieved a greater level of proficiency with the code.[7]

Researchers undertook a similar study when the British Post Office needed to train 10,000 employees to operate new letter sorting machines. In their experiment, four groups of 18 employees, were trained on the new machines: one group trained for one hour a day, the second group trained in two sessions every day, one hour each, the third group trained for one session of two hours every day, while the fourth group trained daily in two sessions of two hours each.

The results of the study confirmed the total time hypothesis, skills improved as a function of time spent, but when you controlled for time the group that trained only for one hour each day outperformed all other groups.[8] This led psychologists to make a distinction between spaced practice and massed practice. In massed practice, someone tries to learn a large amount of material in a short time. Cramming for an exam the next day would be an example of massed practice. Cramming is known to be inefficient and, ultimately, ineffective.[9] Yet it remains a common studying technique.[10] Cramming, of course, could be the result of student trying to organize the demands of school around busy work and social lives, but it also reflects the fact that many students are unaware of the most efficient study techniques.

Cramming also may give a student a false sense of security. In a study titled "when you know that you know and when you think that you know but you don't," researchers projected words one at a time onto a screen. Student volunteers were asked to rate the likelihood that they would remember the words. Later they were given an opportunity to write down as many words as they could remember. This allowed the researchers to compare students' predictions about what they would remember with their actual performance. Some words were repeated and students correctly predicted that they would have better memory for repeated words. However, some words were repeated in close succession and while other word repetitions were spaced out over time. The volunteers predicted that they would have better memory for those words repeated close to each other. In fact, they had better memory for the spaced words. The inescapable conclusion is that cramming gives us an illusion of remembering and may seduce us away from, other, more effective study techniques."

Distinct from massed practice is spaced practice, where material is studied in smaller intervals over a longer period of time. This difference between massed and spaced practice can be seen in two study styles, driven study and balanced study. In driven study, one studies in a few long blocks to the point of exhaustion. This method usually produces poor retention and poor exam performance. Alternatively, if we study in short blocks taking frequent breaks, the balanced approach, we get better retention and better exam performance.[12]

In his delightful essay on memorizing poetry, Jim Holt advised spaced learning:

> ...the key to memorizing a poem painlessly is to do it incrementally, in tiny bits. I knock a couple of new lines into my head each morning before breakfast, hooking them onto what I've already got. At the moment, I'm 22 lines into Tennyson's "Ulysses," with 48 lines to go. It will take me about a month to learn the whole thing at this leisurely pace[13]

Holt's word "leisurely" is important. In education literature, the word memory is often paired with the word rote. Holt points out that "there is torture in the very word 'rote,' which is conjectured to come from the Latin *rota,* meaning 'wheel'."[14] Incremental spaced practice means that memory tasks can be made more enjoyable and more effective.

Why is spacing effective? It could be that the rate memory of consolidation may be limited by some underlying molecular or cellular process and any effort at learning must conform to those base rates.[15] Perhaps, massed practice simply does not allow enough time for these molecular processes to work effectively.[16]

Another plausible explanation for the spacing effect has to do with the level of memory activation. Activation can be thought of as a characteristic of the memory trace that affects accessibility. When activation is high, the memory is easily accessible. When activation is low, the memory is difficult or impossible to retrieve.[17] Conversely, every time we access a memory we increase its level of activation and increase the probability that it can be accessed in the future. Activation decreases with time and increases with repeated exposure. In order to be recalled, a memory must have an activation level greater than some recall threshold. If the activation level falls below the threshold, we may be able to recognize it but not recall it. If it falls even lower, we may not even be able to recognize it. Spaced repetition may strengthen the activation of information in memory.

If you distribute study over time and slowly increase the interval between study sessions, the information is better remembered. This suggests that there may be an optimal distribution of study that would maximize memory.[18] With the correct distribution we could organize study time into relatively small daily sessions. We will see that computer software now allows us to approximate that optimal distribution. Add one more factor, the testing effect, and we will be able to design a powerful memory improvement program.

Ballard's Discovery

The forgetting curve, retention as a declining function of time, is a fundamental feature of memory repeatedly observed since the work of Ebbinghaus. There is however another, much less researched, pattern of retention first observed by Philip Boswood Ballard in 1913. Ballard set out to investigate the claim that slum children had poor memories. To test this assertion he had a group of school boys memorize the poem "On the Loss of the Royal George" by William Cowper. Nineteen boys were given 13 minutes to learn the 36 line poem and were then asked to write as many lines as they could from memory. Only one child could write out the entire poem, while the entire group averaged 27.6 lines.

Two days later Ballard asked the boys to write out the poem again. This was a surprise quiz, he had not told either the boys or their teachers that they would be tested again. This time eight boys wrote out the entire poem and the average performance rose to 30.6 lines. In total, the performance of 16 boys had improved. Most of the boys had recalled lines of poetry on the second test that they could not recall on the first. The other three boys recalled the same number of lines on both tests. In other words most students improved and no student showed a decline in lines remembered. Ballard described these findings as "remarkable" and he repeated the experiment in a number of schools "always with the same result."[9]

On the face of it, these results seemed to contradict the findings of Ebbinghaus. There seemed to be some force at work here that counteracted the forgetting curve. Unfortunately, even though these results were well replicated and demanded explanation, they were largely forgotten or ignored. Many academic books on memory make no mention of Ballard's work.

Interest in Ballard's discovery was re-ignited decades later by psychologist Mathew Erdelyi, who called the phenomenon hypermnesia.[20]

In 1978 Erdelyi published a study, coauthored with Jeff Kleinbard, in which Kleinbard served as the subject. Kleinbard was shown 40 pictures of single objects. The pictures were presented one at a time for five seconds each. After seeing the pictures, Kleinbard was given five minutes to write a list all the pictures he had seen on a sheet with 40 spaces. The list was collected, and Kleinbard was given another sheet and another five minutes to write in the objects he had seen. In effect he was being tested on the list of objects a second time. He was tested in this way five times and each testing interval was five minutes.

For the next week, every time Kleinbard felt like it, he took five minutes to fill in the 40 blanks on a sheet. Once the five minutes were up he sealed the sheet in an envelope and did not review it.

On his first test, he only remembered 19 items, by the time of his final test, 140 hours later, he remembered 36 items. His performance had increased from 48% to 90%. Just like Ballard's school children Kleinbard's performance had improved over time. Kleinbard exhibited hypermnesia and not the forgetting found by Ebbinghaus.[21]

What can account for hypermnesia? Why do these

experiments show less forgetting over time while Ebbinghaus found more? We need to think carefully about the differences between the two experiments. After Ebbinghaus learned a list, he waited some length of time and then tested himself. Remember that his measure of remembering was how long it took him to relearn the list. Once he tested himself on a list over some time period, he could not use that list again. His forgetting curve represents the statistical consolidation of many different lists, each studied once, and each relearned once.

In the hypermnesia experiment, the same list is tested repeatedly. These findings appear to be a special case of the testing effect, the fact that *repeated testing promotes memory.*[22]

The Testing Effect.

Students hate tests and in our era of high stakes testing, testing is almost always seen in a negative light. Most academic testing is done for assessment, to see if a student has mastered a body of knowledge or a set of skills. But testing has other, often forgotten, functions. For example, testing can provide valuable feedback and reinforcement to students and their instructors. One problem with our high stakes testing regime is that it provides information on the scales preferred by policy makers, not on the scales that are most helpful to students. Students need minute to minute feedback, which allows for error correction and reinforcement of target information. An infrequent high stakes test is a source of anxiety for students and the information that it provides comes much too late. The shame of this is that we know that frequent low stakes, low anxiety, testing with immediate feedback improves memory.

Psychologist Fred Keller discovered this principle while trying to design an optimal method for teaching Morse code during World War II. He invented the code-voice teaching method. Here he describes the approach:

> I would sound a signal with my key: about three seconds later I would announce the signal's name — the letter or digit; in the time between the signal and the voice, my pupil would try to print the appropriate character on a sheet of paper. If he succeeded, the announcement presumably reinforced his action; if he failed, it told him of his error. . . The aim of the procedure was threefold: (1) to encourage the student to react to ever signal of the code when it was sent; (2) to provide immediate reinforcement for each correct response; and (3) to determine the nature of every error made. The procedure permitted the individual student to move to a higher level of training as soon as he showed that he was ready to do so.[23]

Behavior analyst Julie Vargas reminds us that immediate feedback should be delivered before the next question or task is begun. She points out "a student who adds 19 and 21 and gets 211 needs help right away not after completing a whole paper of similar incorrectly added numbers."[24] This type of testing is of real benefit to the student and is the antithesis of the high stakes testing approach that dominates American education.

Testing helps memory through feedback and

reinforcement, but the hypermnesia experiments suggest that there must be an additional factor in play. Remember that in these experiments no feedback was provided. Simply giving another test produced improvement. Clearly the information was still in long term memory, but some reason it could not be accessed for the first test. In addition, when accessed on a subsequent test, the memory for the information became stronger. One explanation for this testing effect is retrieval practice. The act of retrieval may itself strengthen a memory.

The spacing and testing effect seem to be closely related to each other. The retrieval required by testing is in itself a learning event, in effect a repetition, and if the retrieval is carefully spaced to occur before the memory fails, then the original memory is strengthened.[25]

Harnessing the Spacing and Testing Effects

Basic science discovers underlying principles and often we are able to use our knowledge of those principles to make some improvement in the world. In medicine, for example, our knowledge of the cause of disease has led to treatments and cures. There is no reason the same should not apply to the scientific study of memory. Over the years there have been a number of successful applications of the spacing and testing effect to improve memory.

Paul Pimsleur

"Probably no aspect of learning a foreign language is more important than memory. A student must remember several thousand words and a considerable number of processes for adapting and combining them to attain even a minimal proficiency." — Paul Pimsleur[26]

You may have heard of the popular Pimsleur language programs. Paul Pimsleur was a professor of education and romance languages who designed the first computerized language laboratory.[27]

Pimsleur argued that memory was the most important part of language learning. According to Pimsleur "to become a fairly fluent speaker of a language, with 5,000 words at his command, a person would have to learn ten new words a day, day in and day out, for a year and a half."[28] Pimsleur blamed poor language teaching for the fact "that an overwhelming majority of language students do quit at the earliest possible moment"[29] He tried to harness insights from memory science to improve language instruction.

Pimsleur realized that the curve of forgetting must apply to language learning. Most new material is forgotten soon after the first presentation. Thus, new material should be studied again soon after initial learning. As memories consolidate the space between repetitions could be increased.

By presenting students with frequent reviews of material spaced over time, he could alter the slope of the forgetting curve. One can see this principle at work by listening to one of Pimsleur's language program. Pimsleur presented material according to an exponential scale. A vocabulary word might be repeated 5 seconds after first being introduced. The term would then presented again at 25 seconds, and then at 125 seconds, and so on. By the fourth repetition, the interval has expanded to ten minutes and by the eight the repetition the interval is five days.[30]

Pimsleur noted that attempts to teach vocabulary words in a specific order would suffer from the serial position effect. Students would have better memory for the first and last words and be more likely to forget words in the middle of the list. To overcome this, he argued that there must be some degree of randomization in the repeated presentation of words.

Pimsleur language programs are often available in the public library and I encourage you to try one.

Spaced Retrieval in the Treatment of Dementia

Space retrieval has been used successfully to teach new information to patients with Alzheimer's disease. A typical use of the technique it to teach the patient the name of a caregiver. The patient is asked to repeat the caregiver's name after an interval of 15 seconds. If the response is successful, the interval is doubled to 30 seconds then to 1, 2, 3, 8, 16, and 32 minutes. If the patient fails to recall the name, the caregiver gives the name again and returns to the last interval for the last successful attempt.[31]

SQ3R, PQRST, and 3R

These acronyms, SQ3R, PQRST, and 3R, are more than just an alphabet soup. They are the names given to techniques for solving a familiar problem, the fact that most students do not study effectively. Surveys reveal that the two most common study strategies are taking notes from the assigned reading, and rereading the textbook and classroom notes. While these approaches do involve repetition, they do not provide students with feedback or retrieval practice.[32]

We know that the forgetting curve applies to academic material. In one famous study a group of students was tested immediately after reading text. They retained 53% of the material they had just read. Another group of students was tested two weeks after reading the same text. They remembered only 20%.

Simple repetition, re-reading the text, did help counteract the effects of forgetting. After one immediate rereading, average retention rose from 53% to 74%. Ohio State University, psychologist Francis Robinson wanted to know if there was "some other more efficient method of studying than reading and reading a lesson."[33] In addition, if such a method could be discovered could it be taught?

The idea that students need direct instruction in study skill is not new. In 1914, Latin and Greek teacher T. B. Glass complained "that the average student does not know how to study." [34] Unfortunately, much of the early literature on study strategy was shaped by anecdote and philosophical speculation. This begins to change in the 1920s as colleges introduced how-to-study classes. By the 1940s, educational psychologists had come to realize the importance of skill instruction. It had become clear that people who taught themselves (as many did at one time) swimming or typing did not perform as well as those who received instruction. Robinson believed that what was true for typing and swimming must also be true for studying. Most students are self taught in study techniques and the methods they use are often ineffective. Students needed to learn how to learn.

But what to teach them? Here Robinson turned to experimental psychology to find new approaches. Using research findings, he developed a study technique called SQ3R.

SQ3R is a mnemonic for Survey Question Read Recall Review. When a student approaches a text to study, say an assigned book chapter, the first step is to survey. The student should glance over the chapter to see what the main points are and read the chapter headings. If there is a summary paragraph, then that should also be read. This process should take about a minute and give the student a sense of the major ideas.

The second step is to question. Here the student looks at the first heading in the chapter and turns it into a question.

Now the student reads that first section of the chapter, trying to answer the question. This way reading becomes more of an active process. After reading that section, the student puts the book aside and tries to recite an answer to the question. The student now goes back and questions, reads, and recites for each successive headed section.

When all the sections are completed, the student reviews then reviews the entire chapter, using the student generated questions as a check on understanding.[35]

A similar approach is named PQRST, Preview Question Read State Test.[36] The benefits of these methods are not confined to students, in one study of adults over the age of 50 PQRST was shown to improve memory.[37]

However, while SQ3R and PQRST have been shown to be effective, they are needlessly complex. A simpler alternative is 3R. 3R stands for Read, Recite, and Read.

In 3R students first reads the text and, then, after putting the text down, recites as much as they can remember from their reading. After the recitation, they reread the text. According to researchers, 3R is easier to teach and learn than other study strategies. It requires less work on the part of students. In addition, because it involves retrieval, it engages the testing effect, which, as we have shown, improves memory. It also provides feedback, allowing students to gauge their knowledge. The final reading provides repetition and students are able to check their answers.

In several experiments, researchers found that students using 3R outperformed students using only note taking and rereading. They did so with less total study time. Not only did 3R improve retention it also improved performance on problem solving tests.[38] Once again we see that better memory does not hurt higher order skills, such as problem solving. If you want to improve higher order thinking, better memory is an important prerequisite.

The inventors of 3R suggest that students could recite material (the second R) while exercising. This suggestion is remarkably similar to a technique used by Alexander Arguelles to study foreign languages. Arguelles is a scholar who can read dozens of languages. He calls this technique shadowing. It consists of walking fast while reciting language learning material.[39] Arguelles also advocates another technique similar to 3R he calls scriptorium. The scriptorium technique consists of reading a sentence out loud in the language you wish to learn, writing it down, and then reading it out loud from your writing. He explains the technique in more detail at his website: foreignlanguageexpertise.com. While shadowing and the scriptorium method have not been scientifically evaluated, they both seem engage the same processes as the 3R technique.

The observation that learning can improve while walking is not unique to Arguelles. Psychologist Seth Roberts made a similar observation and found, through self-experimentation, that his Chinese language learning improved during treadmill walking.[40]

Flash Cards

I have already mentioned Fred Keller's work on Morse code learning. In the course of describing his work, Keller tells this illuminating anecdote about one of his students, Richard Youtz:

> On his first practice runs his error scores were large, and typical, but on the next evening, at his second training session, he made no errors at all. For a very good reason; on one side of 36 cards he had pictured a basic signal, in dot-dash form; on the other he had written the matching letter or digit; at spare moments throughout the day, he would look at the dots and dashes, *whistle* their pattern, and guess at

the names before checking. He taught me more than the students who followed the rules.[41]

Credit for the invention of flashcards has often been erroneously assigned to Favell Lee Mortimer. According to this story, she first presented them in her 1857 book *Reading Without Tears or a Pleasant Mode of Learning to Read*. Ms. Mortimer is most famous for a series of children's geography books that described nations she never visited in unflattering stereotypes. For example, she described the people of Italy as "ignorant and wicked" and wrote that the Greeks "love singing, though they sing badly."[42]

It is clear, however, that flashcards predated the work of the ill-tempered Ms. Mortimer. John Stuart Mill speaks of his father writing out Greek vocabulary cards for him around 1809.[43] Educational playing cards were invented by the Franciscan Monk Thomas Murner in the 16th century. However, these do not appear, to have been flashcards. The cards carried educational and mnemonic images on their faces, so that students could learn while they played. It is claimed that his students progressed so rapidly using these cards that Murner was initially accused of magic.[44]

The earliest example of true flashcards that I could find was a proposal made by theologian Issac Watts in 1751. Watts suggested that children could be taught using double-sided cards:

May not some little tablets of pasteboard be made in imitation of cards which might teach the unlearned several parts of grammar, philosophy, geometry, geography, astronomy, &c.

What if one side of these tablets or charts, a town or city were named or described; and on the other side, of the country, province, kingdom, where that town stands; with some geographical or historical remark on it; and whosoever in play draws the chart with the town on it, should be obliged to tell country where it stands, and the remark made on it?

Watts even describes the use of the cards for foreign language study: "or if one side were a word in English: and on the other the same thing expressed in Latin, Greek, or French for those who learn these languages."[45]

Flashcards are effective because they employ several important principles of memory consolidation, including repetition, and the testing effect. They also help students with comprehension monitoring. Students frequently use repetition to study. For example, they will read a textbook passage over and over again. Many students, however, seem averse to testing themselves. They often will not complete the practice questions at the end of the chapter or quiz themselves on the material.

The failure to self quiz means that students not only forgo the benefits of the testing effect, they also set themselves up for the illusion of knowing. Students may walk into the exam thinking they know the material, but under perform on the test. Frequent rereading, while it can improve memory, it can also give a false sense of knowing the material. This belief is called the illusion of knowing.

The student complaint, "I studied hard but did poorly on the exam," often reflects a failure to monitor comprehension. If you test yourself with flash cards or computer software or have someone else quiz you, you will experience not only the benefits of the testing effect, but also receive feedback about your areas of strength and weakness. You will, in effect, learn what you know and what you don't know and apportion your study time more effectively.[46]

Unfortunately many students who use flashcards do not use them effectively. The practice of setting aside cards that the student knows may contribute to forgetting. While it seems reasonable that dropping a known card allows more time to study more difficult cards, research suggests students often drop cards prematurely, after a single successful recall. The assumption that the information is well learned is often mistaken, and the student may forget the material.[47] In other words, if the known cards are kept in the pack, the additional review will increase resistance to forgetting.

It is also a mistake to review flashcards in the same order. When we try to memorize a list, we have better memory for the items at the beginning and the end. This phenomenon is called the serial order effect. If you try to recall the lyrics to a song, you will often discover that you have better memory for words at the beginning and the end than you do for the words in the middle. This effect generalizes to many lists, for example, when asked to recall the names of US presidents volunteers had good memory for the first few presidents and the most recent, but, with the exception of Abraham Lincoln, poor memory for the presidents in between. [48] Similarly if you keep reviewing flashcards in the same order you might have poorer memory for the cards in the middle of the pack.

Another reason to shuffle flashcards is that the position of a card may become a cue for identity of other cards. If you know that a card falls in a certain order, you may be forming an association between the information and its position in the deck. Since in other contexts, such as on an exam, the order cues will not be available, we do not want to become dependent on them. Thus, flashcards are more effective if you shuffle them frequently.

Flash cards are good, but we can make them more effective. An example of a well thought out strategy for flash card use is called SAFMEDS: Say All Fast in a Minute Everyday Shuffled. The SAFMEDS approach was designed to help students develop automaticity in the basic skills, such as number facts. A typical card might have a math problem on one side, for example, 7 X 8. The correct answer, in this case 56, would appear on the reverse side. The goal is to answer correctly as many possible in a minute. As you work through the deck, you give your answer and check it by looking at the back of the card. Cards are dealt either into a pile of correct and or a pile incorrect responses. This allows the learner to calculate the proportion of correct responses. The cards are shuffled every day to eliminate any reliance on serial order effects.

An important component of SAFMEDS is record keeping. Daily results are recorded and charted so that you can see your progress. This highlights daily improvement, which can have a motivating effect.[49]

SAFMEDS employs many important principles

from learning theory. It provides for daily, that is spaced, practice. It gives immediate feedback, that is, you learn right away the correct answer. It is limited in time, one minute a day, and, thus, practice does not become aversive.

One other memory principle that can be employed with flash cards is the use of visual imagery. You can use pictures as well as words. Research has shown that foreign language vocabulary flashcards are more effective if they associate a picture with a noun, rather than the English word.[50]

From Index Cards to Computers

Science journalist Sebastian Leitner invented a flash card system that attempted to maximize the effects of distributed practice and the testing effect. He called his system, which consisted of nothing more than flashcards and a divided card file, the hand computer.[51] Higbee describes a simplified version of the hand computer that he used to memorize scripture:

> I used an increasing-interval review schedule during a 16-month period when I was memorizing scriptures. I learned one new scripture each day, and carried with me seven scriptures on cards – the new one I was learning that day plus the six I had learned the previous six days. After seven days, a card would go into a file to be reviewed once a week for a month, then once a month for several months, and then once every three months. The schedule of gradually increasing intervals helped me to memorize about 500 scriptures (averaging about two verses each) in

16 months.[52]

Improved versions of these techniques have been now been incorporated into computer flashcard software. Daily use of these programs allows us to optimize the power of spaced repetition and the testing effect. You choose the information you wish to remember and create a set of virtual flashcards. For every card, an assessment is made for how well you know that information. If you do not know it at all, you be asked about it again after a short wait, perhaps the next day. If the fact is well known, you will see it much less often.

I am aware of at least three excellent software packages for this type of memory improvement: Supermemo, Mnemosyne, and Anki. Of these, my preference is Anki, a program originally designed for learning the Japanese Kanji script, but adaptable for a variety of learning tasks. Anki, which means memorizing in Japanese, is easy to use and is available for download at http://ankisrs.net/

Every day Anki selects a number of cards to test you on. After you attempt a response, the software informs you of the correct answer and you rate how easy or difficult it was to remember the information. Your choices are "again" (if you could not remember at all), "hard," "easy" and "very easy." Based on your rating Anki will schedule the next appearance of the card. If the card was difficult and you did not remember it at all, the card will be scheduled again very soon, either in the current session or the next day's. If was very easy to recall the software will schedule the next test in the future, days, months, or even years away. Thus, the software gives you the benefits of the testing effect, immediate feedback, and the spacing effect.

Anki flashcards are organized into decks. You can either create your own deck or download one from a growing list of decks created by Anki users and posted on the Anki website. There are decks available for a wide range of topics, including many languages and academic subjects.

If you choose to download an existing deck, I recommend changing the Anki settings to reduce the number of new cards it presents every day. If the number is too high, you may be overwhelmed and frustrated by the number of cards you don't know. Mastering a few new cards a day is easier and more reinforcing.

However, I also recommend, when possible, that you create your own deck rather than use an existing one. Notice that I said deck and not decks. You are better off with a single deck covering many topics that interest you than separate decks for each topic. This way you are not tempted to skip some subjects. In addition, single subject decks may give unintended cues or have serial position effects that could slow your development of fluency.

It is easy to store your deck online, either through the Anki website, or on a computer cloud service such as Dropbox or on the Anki server. This way you can access your cards from a variety of platforms, including home and office computers and smartphones.

In Anki, each card is defined as a question and answer pair. Cards can be set up so that one is always designated as the question and other, the correct response. Alternatively, using the backwards/forwards option you will be sometimes be presented with one side of the card and sometimes presented with the other. The backwards/forward option is useful in foreign language learning. Sometimes you would be asked to translate from English to the target language, other times you would be asked to translate into English.

When I use Anki for learning foreign language vocabulary, I enter a word in English on one side and the foreign language equivalent on the other. After each word I put, in parentheses, the name of the target language. So one side might read "amiko (English)" and the other side would be "friend (Esperanto)." Thus, using the forward/backwards option, I would sometimes be asked to translate from English to Esperanto other times I would move from Esperanto to English.

If I wanted to remember the title of a movie, on the forward card, I might write a description the film. For example, "Martin Scorsese film about an orphan and his automaton living in a Paris train station." The answer card would read *Hugo*. Since we often forget the titles of movies but remember the plots, I always make it a point to add a card to Anki for every new film I see.

We often forget book titles and the names of their authors. Here I use the forward/backwards feature of Anki. I create a card with the name of the author and one with the book title. Each side of the card includes a word in parentheses indicating the type of answer needed. For example, one side might read "*Learn to*

Remember (author)." The other side might read "Dominic O'Brien (book)." Using the forward/backwards feature, sometimes Anki will ask for the name of the author, expecting to be answered with the name of the book. Other times Anki will ask for the name of the book. Learning the names of the books I have read helps me remember their contents. People are often unduly impressed that I can name the titles and authors of so many books. It is not because my memory is any better than anyone else's, it is because I spend 5 to 10 minutes a day using Anki.

We can combine techniques and use Anki to learn mnemonics. For example, if I want to learn how many feet there in a mile (5,280) I use the word in I created in the Dominic System (explained in Chapter 7) that encodes this information (EBHO). Then I create a question that reads "Dominic word for feet in a mile." The answer is, of course, "EBHO." After I have learned the mnemonic, I might, then, create a separate question: how many feet are there in a mile? After I have learned the mnemonic, I would have no trouble answering the question directly. When I felt comfortable enough with the direct question, I could even delete the mnemonic card from the deck.

Anki will also accept pictures and sound files. You could enter a photo of someone whose name you wish to remember or a piece of art so you can memorize the artist's name. Forget the name of a movie star? Find the celebrity's picture on Google Images and copy and paste it onto an Anki card.

Using Anki to Reduce Tip of Tongue Forgetting

I have devised a strategy to use Anki against tip of the tongue states and other memory failures. The guiding assumption here is that tip of the tongue states are indicators of areas of memory weakness. The fact that tip of the tongue states often recur for the same words suggests that there is some weakness in our ability to access that piece of information or in the strength of the memory trace itself. Alternatively it could be a case of interference, where one memory interferes with the recall of another. In order to overcome tip of the tongue states, we must increase the activation of a memory and strengthen its association with other ideas.

Like pain to the athlete, tip of the tongue states point us to areas of concern. If we cannot recall some fact, there is a good chance that we will have trouble with that same fact in the future. A tip of the tongue state is a warning, it alerts us that we need to strengthen that memory. Our first step is to keep a record of our tip of the tongue memory lapses. Perhaps it sounds contradictory, but we must remember our forgetting. I used to carry in my pocket a small memo book where I would try to record all my tip of the tongue forgetting. Now I use note taking software on my smartphone. I use the Wunderlist application which synchronizes with a list maintained on my computer, making it is very easy to copy and paste the information to Anki.

If I forget the name of the lead singer of the band KISS (Gene Simmons) or the name of the 33rd president (Harry Truman), it goes onto my list. I try to write down the tip of the tongue state as soon as possible after it occurs. I write it down whether I have recovered the information or not. If I cannot recall the answer, I will write down what little I remember and look it up later. It is certainly true that there are marvelous sources of information available on the internet, but I do not stop with satisfying my curiosity or resolving the anxiety of not knowing the answer. Lapses in memory are evidence of weakened or weakening associations. By identifying and addressing these our forgetting, we can strengthen the brain's network of associations. Entering it into Anki reduces the probability that I will have the same memory lapse in the future. A few minutes every day with Anki will strengthen the information in your memory and improve your chances of recalling it in the future. In addition, as I have pointed out earlier, learning and retaining more facts improves our memory by making it easier to form new mental associations.

Another approach to tip of the tongue forgetting is to strengthen the link between the blocking information and the information you want to recall. Psychologist James Weinland gives the example of the name Rheingold interfering with recall of the name Rheinweld. Here one could create a mnemonic "gold can be welded, and Rheingold can bring up Rheinweld."[53] This way the blocking information can be turned into a cue for the desired information. These mnemonics can be entered into Anki to ensure that they are well learned.

Daily use of Anki is a highly effective way to train your memory, to build up you knowledge base and create more associative hooks where you can hang other memories. the commitment of time is minimal, but the rewards are great. Forget less and remember more, these are yours with a commitment to short daily practice.

Make Memory Training a Priority

Of course, memory training cannot be your only priority, but it should be *a* priority. For this system to work, you need to spend a few minutes a day using the software. The demands of daily life may tend to push out your memory practice. Physician and stress expert Edward Charlesworth's simple message, "if you are too busy to exercise, you are too busy"[54] is also true for memory exercise. Put your memory training on your calendar and commit to these few moments every day.

The Future of Memory Training

Anki and other memory improvement programs are just the beginning. New artificial intelligence programs are being created that will make memory training easier and more enjoyable.

To understand why this might be the case, let us examine an example of human skills improved by the use of computers. In the past few decades, the average age of chess grandmasters has been falling. In 1950, the youngest chess grandmaster was a 26 year old named David Bronstein. By 2002, the youngest grandmaster, Sergey Karjakin, was only 12 years old. Why are children playing better chess now than in the past? Because they practice more often with better opponents, chess playing computers. To become an expert chess player you need to play thousands of game against challenging opponents. Computerized chess gives children the opportunity to play frequently at a very high level. In addition, the computer makes its moves quickly reducing the time for each game and making it possible to play more frequently.

Recently, the military has been testing the Tactical Language Training System. This program uses speech recognition, artificial intelligence, and a game like interface to teach soldiers Arabic. The software places the learner in a simulation which requires basic language skills. The computer monitors progress and optimizes the presentation of new information.[55]

In 1984, educational psychologist Benjamin Bloom noted what he called the two sigma problem in education. In a series of studies, Bloom found that students who received individual tutoring achieved about two standard deviations above students in conventional classrooms.[56] Sigma is the symbol used by statisticians to represent a standard deviation, hence the name two sigma. It is easy to see why individual tutoring is so effective, the tutor can provide both immediate feedback and instruction tailored to the needs of the individual student. The problem, of course, is the cost. As Albert Corbett pointed out "individual human tutoring is the most effective and most expensive form of instruction."[57]

Tutoring software that embodies the principles of memory science is destined to become an important component of education.

---

[1] Bahrick, H. P. (1984). Semantic memory content in

permastore: Fifty years of memory for Spanish Learned in School. *Journal of Experimental Psychology: General, 113,* 1 - 29

[2] Radvansky, G. A. (2011). *Human memory.* Boston; Allyn & Bacon.

[3] Appleton-Knapp, S., Bjork, R. A., & Wickens, T. D. (2005). Examining the spacing effect in advertising: Encoding variability, retrieval processes and their interaction. *Journal of Consumer Research, 32,* 266-276.

[4] Xue, G. et al., (2010). Greater neural pattern similarity across repetitions is associated with better memory. *Science, 330,* 97 – 101.

[5] Baddeley, A. D. (1976). *The psychology of memory.* New York: Basic Books.

[6] King, T. W. (2000). *Modern Morse code in rehabilitation and education.* Boston: Allyn and Bacon.

[7] Woodworth, R. S. & Schlosberg, H. (1954). *Experimental Psychology* (Revised edition). New York: Holt, Reinhart and Winston.

[8] Baddeley, A. D. (1976). *The psychology of memory.* New York: Basic Books.

[9] Kornell, N. (2009). Optimising learning using flashcards: Spacing is more effective than cramming. *Applied Cognitive Psychology, 23,* 1297–1317

[10] Donovan, C., Figlio, D. N, & Rush, M.(2006).

Cramming: The effects of school accountability on college-bound students. (Working Paper 12628). Cambridge, MA: Nationl Bureau of Economic Research.

[11] Zechmeister, E. B. & Shaughnessy, J. J. (1980). When you know that you know and when you think that you know buy you don't. *Bulletin of the Psychonomic Society, 15,* 41 -44.

[12] Powell, R. A., Symbaluk, D. G., & Honey, P. L. (2009). *Introduction to learning and behavior.* 3rd Ed. Belmont, CA: Warsworth.

[13] Holt, J. (April 5, 2009). Got poetry? *The New York Times.* (p. BR23)

[14] Holt, J. (April 5, 2009). Got poetry? *The New York Times.* (p. BR23)

[15] Baddeley, A. D. (1976). *The psychology of memory.* New York: Basic Books.

[16] Nation, I.S. P. (2001). *Learning vocabulary in another language.* Cambridge, UK: Cambridge University Press.

[17] Baddeley, A., Eysenck, M. W., & Anderson, M. C. (2010). *Memory.* New York: Psychology Press.

[18] Cepeda, N. J, et al (2009). Optimizing distributed practice: Theoretical analysis and practical implications. *Experimental Psychology, 56,* 236 – 246.

[19] Ballard, P. B. (1913). *Obliviscence and Reminiscence.*

Cambridge, UK: Cambridge University Press. (p.. 2).

[20] Erdelyi, M. H. (1996). *The rediscovery of unconscious memories.* Chicago: The University of Chicago Press.

[21] Erdelyi, M. H., , & Kleinbard, J. (1978). Has Ebbinghaus decayed with time? The growth of recall (hypermnesia) over days. *Journal of Experimental Psychology: Human Learning & Memory, 4,* 275-289.

[22] Wheeler, M. A. & Roediger, H. L. (1992). Disparate effects of repeated testing: Reconciling Ballard's (1913) and Bartlett's (1932) results. *Psychological Science, 3,* 240 - 245.

[23] Keller, F. S. (1979). *Summers and sabbaticals; Selected papers on psychology and education. Champaign,* IL: Research Press. (pp. 28 - 29).

[24] Vargas, J. S. (2009). *Behavior analysis for effective teaching.* New York: Routledge. (p. 195).

[25] Appleton-Knapp, S., Bjork, R. A., & Wickens, T. D. (2005). Examining the spacing effect in advertising: Encoding variability, retrieval processes and their interaction. *Journal of Consumer Research, 32,* 266-276.

[26] Pimsleur, P. (1967). A memory schedule. *The Modern Language Journal, 51,* 73 - 75. (p. 73).

[27] Paul Pimsleur, 48, dies in France. (1976, June 29). New York Times, p. 34.

[28] Pimsleur, P. (1980). *How to learn a foreign language.* Boston: Heinle & Heinle Publishers. (p. 61).

[29] Pimsleur, P. (1980). *How to learn a foreign language.* Boston: Heinle & Heinle Publishers. (p. 28).

[30] Nation, I.S. P. (2001). *Learning vocabulary in another language.* Cambridge, UK: Cambridge University Press.

[31] Broman, M. (2001). Space retrieval: A behavioral approach to memory improvement I Alzheimer's and related dementias. *NYS Psychologist, 13,* 31 – 34.

[32] Dunlosky, J., Rawson, K. A., Marsh, E. J., Nathan, M. J., & Willingham, D. T. (2013). Improving students' learning with effective learning techniques promising directions from cognitive and educational psychology. *Psychological Science in the Public Interest, 14*(1), 4-58.

[33] Robinson, F. (1961). *Effective study: Revised edition.* New York: Harper & Brothers. (p. 14)

[34] Glass, T. B. (1914). Suggestions for teaching students how to study Latin and Greek. *The Classical Weekly, 8,* (6), 43 - 45. (p. 43).

[35] Robinson, F. (1961). *Effective study: Revised edition.* New York: Harper & Brothers.

[36] Wormeli, R. (2005) *Summarization in any subject: 50 techniques to improve student learning.* Alexandria, VA: Association for Supervision and Curriculum Development.

[37] West, R. L., Bagwell, D. K., & Dark-Freudeman, A.(2008). Self-Efficacy and Memory Aging: The Impact of a Memory Intervention Based on Self-Efficacy. *Aging, Neuropsychology & Cognition, 15,* 302-329.

[38] McDaniel, , M. A., Howard, D. C., and Einstein, G. O., (2009). The read-recite-review study strategy: Effective and portable. *Psychological Science, 20,* 516 - 522.

[39] Erard, M. (2012). *Babel no more: The search for the world's most extraordinary language learners.* New York: Free Press.

[40] Roberts, S. D. (2014). How Little We Know: Big Gaps in Psychology and Economics. *International Journal of Comparative Psychology, 27*(2), 190 - 203.

[41] Keller, F. S. (1979). *Summers and sabbaticals; Selected papers on psychology and education. Champaign,* IL: Research Press. (p. 29).

[42] Pruzan, T. & Mortimer, F. L. (2005). *The clumsiest people in Europe or: Mrs. Mortimer's bad tempered guide to the Victorian world.* New York: Bloomsbury Publishing. (p. 54, p. 87).

[43] Mill, J. S. (1957/1873). *Autobiography.* Indianapolis, IN: Bobbs-Merrill Educational Publishing.

[44] Hargrave, C. P. (1966). *A history of playing cards and a bibliography of cards and gaming.* New York: Dover Publications.

[45] Watts, I. (1832/1751). *The improvement of the mind:*

to which is added a discourse on the education of children and youth. New York: Betts & Anstice. (pp. 303 - 304, p. 304).

[46] Glenberg, A. M., Wilkinson, A. C., & Epstein, W. (1982). The illusion of knowing: Failure in the self-assessment of comprehension. *Memory & Cognition, 10*(6), 597-602.

[47] Kornell, N., & Bjork, R. A. (2008). Optimizing self-regulated study: The benefits – and costs – of dropping flashcards. *Memory, 16*, 125 – 136.

[48] Roediger, H. L. & Crowder, R. G. (1976). A serial position effect in recall of United States Presidents. *Bulletin of the Psychonomic Society, 8*, 275 - 278.

[49] Vargas, J. S. (2009). *Behavior analysis for effective teaching.* New York: Routledge.

[50] Weber, N. E. (1978). Pictures and words as stimuli in learning foreign language responses. *The Journal of Psychology, 96*, 57 – 63.

[51] Mondria, J. & Vries, S. M. (1993). Efficiently memorizing words with the help of word cards and "hand computer": Theory and application. *System, 22*, 47 -57.

[52] Higbee, K. L. (2001). *Your memory: How it works and how to improve it.* New York: Marlowe & Company. (pp. 89 - 90)

[53] Weinland, J. D. (1957). *How to improve your memory.* New York: Barnes and Noble, Inc. (p. 45).

[54] Charlesworth, E. A. & Nathan, R. G. (1985). *Stress*

management: A comprehensive guide to wellness. New York: Ballantine books. (p. 337).

[55] Johnson, W. L. (2010).Serious use of a serious game for language learning. *International Journal of Artificial Intelligence in Education, 20,* 175-195

[56] Bloom, B. S. (1984). The 2 sigma problem: the search for methods of group instruction as effective as one-to-one tutoring. *Educational Researcher, 13,* 4-16.

[57] Corbett, A. (2001). Cognitive computer tutors: Solving the two-sigma problem. In M. Bauer, P. Gmytrasiewicz, & J. Vassileva (Eds.), *UM2001, User Modeling: Proceedings of the Eighth International Conference* (pp. 137–147). Berlin: Springer.

Chapter 10

Other Memory Improvement Techniques

In this chapter I will briefly describe several other memory techniques that have been shown to be effective.

Memrise

An adjunct or possible an alternative to Anki for learning foreign language vocabulary and other material is the web service Memrise. Memrise was developed by memory champion Ed Cooke. The website has a clever user interface that allows you to add new words at your own pace and gives you daily practice that takes advantage of the testing and spacing effect. Dozens of languages and academic subjects are available. Language learners would be well advised to take advantage of this service. The web address is http://www.memrise.com/

Mind Maps and Memory

Mind mapping is a technique invented by Tony Buzan. A mind map is a graphic representation of associated information. The major subject is in a central oval and branches representing important themes radiate out from this center. The map serves as an alternative to standard note taking and outlining as a method of organizing and studying information. Buzan claims that mind maps better represent the way information is stored in the brain. By extension, he argues that when you create a mind map your brain will better grasp and remember the information it represents.

While some of Buzan's claims for mind mapping seem extravagant, there is evidence that the technique has value. Researchers have found when students construct a graphic representation of information, comprehension and memory are enhanced.[1] Mind mapping bears some resemblance to the method of loci and it seems that the spatial arrangement of information does improve retention. It may also be that the drawing creates artificial spatial cues that improve memory beyond the purely semantic cues found in the information.[2]

You can learn this technique from *The Mind Map Book* by Tony Buzan.[3]

Sleep and Memory

A review of Ebbinghaus's work suggested that memory for nonsense syllables was better if sleep intervened between learning and testing. Subsequent research has shown this is a robust effect, if we sleep immediately after learning, our memory of the information is improved. Two hypotheses have emerged to explain this observation. One, the interference hypothesis, suggests forgetting is often the consequence of new information interfering with the formation of memories. The idea here is that if we learn something just before sleep, we are more likely to remember it because sleep protects the memory from new interfering information.

An alternative is the consolidation hypothesis which asserts that one of the functions of sleep is to consolidate information in the long term memory. According to this hypothesis during sleep our brains engage in an active process that helps consolidate information in long term memory.

Current evidence seems to support the sleep-memory-consolidation hypothesis. We know now that there are different stages of sleep. If the interference hypothesis were true, we would expect all stages to have the same effect on memory, since all stages prevent interfering sensory inputs. This is not the case, the sleep stage does matter.[4] Slow brain wave sleep enhances declarative memory while rapid eye movement sleep enhances procedural memory. This is consistent with other findings; we know that hormone cortisol and neurotransmitter acetylcholine interfere with declarative memory. During slow wave sleep the levels of cortisol and acetylcholine are reduced, suggesting that declarative memory consolidation will be superior while in this state.[5]

Backward chaining

Backwards chaining is a technique where sequenced material, such as a list or a poem, is learned in reverse order. The last step is learned first. Generally, when we learn new material we work from the beginning until we hit a difficult spot. Then we start from the beginning and work through to that spot again. One problem with this is that our anxiety increases as we get closer to the difficult part. In backwards chaining, we learn the end first. That way we are always moving towards a section we have already mastered. This reduces anxiety because the task becomes easier as we move towards the end.[6]

Elaboration

There are different ways to pack a suitcase. Airline employees and frequent travelers often become expert at packing their carry on luggage. In memory, it also matters how it is packed. We can see this in a strange phenomenon called the Baker baker paradox. In memory experiments, people are more likely to remember that someone's occupation is a baker than they are to remember a person's name is Baker. In this case, even though the word is identical, one taps into a deep web of associations the other doesn't.[7]

Information is stored in long term memory through a process of association. We forge bonds of association between new information and existing knowledge. The active creation of these connections is called elaboration. Inventing mnemonics is a kind of elaboration, but the process is broader than this. It includes actively looking for meaning in new material. If you are able to find meaning in information, you will better remember it.

Meditation

I first discovered meditation as a young teenager when I came across a paperback yoga book in a drugstore rack. I didn't know anything about yoga, few did back then, but I was always interested in new ideas, so I bought the book. I remember that it advised sitting meditation as a way to relax, and I found this seemed to relieve the frequent headaches I had as a child.

With age and scientific training, I now have sufficient detachment to be skeptical of my own experience. Childhood memories are often inaccurate and people are predisposed to see correlations where none exist. Just as I cannot draw firm conclusions from other people's anecdotal stories I must practice the same vigilance towards my own. We must be prepared to follow the advice of physicist Richard Feynman, "the first principle is that you must not fool yourself , and you are the easiest person to fool."[8]

There have been many anecdotal accounts claiming that yoga in general and meditation in particular improves memory. Some of these accounts are quite ancient. There is, for example, in Hinduism the claim that the practice of personal restraint allowed ancient sages to pass on the sacred Vedic texts with perfect fidelity before the invention of writing.[9]

Scientific evidence has been more elusive. Indeed, one large scale meta-analysis of meditation research concluded that many studies have been plagued with methodological problems and that the evidence for meditation's benefits was in fact quite weak.[10] To see why this might be the case let us look at a 2009 study conducted by Ellen Luders and her colleagues.

The researchers recruited 22 long term meditation practitioners (5 to 46 years) and took high resolution magnetic resonance images of their brains. For a comparison group 22 brain scans matched for age, gender, and education were drawn from an existing data base. They found significant structural differences between the two groups. The meditators had larger gray matter volumes for several brain areas including the right hippocampus. Since the hippocampus is involved in the formation of long term memories, this suggests that meditation might contribute to an improved memory.[11]

These results are intriguing. Unfortunately, this study does not allow us to form a strong conclusion. The problem is that we do not know what the brains of the meditators looked like before they started daily meditation. It is completely plausible that their brains differed from the comparison group even before they took up meditation. Perhaps someone with more gray matter in the hippocampus is more likely to practice meditation. The procedure used in this study could not rule out this alternative explanation.

This does not mean that the study was pointless. It suggests that meditation might cause important physical changes to the brain. It is suggestive but not definitive. At minimum, it tells us this might be a promising area for research.

Fortunately, a number of studies have made a more convincing case for the cognitive benefits of meditation. For example, one study, conducted by Kam-Tim So and David Orme-Johnson, looked at the effects of Transcendental Meditation on Taiwanese high school students. The students were randomly assigned to the treatment or control groups and were measured before and after the experiment. The advantage of the random assignment is that it eliminates the possibility that meditators might be a self-selected group possessing cognitive or biological characteristics not shared by non-meditators.

The researchers found that those assigned to the meditation group improved their performance on a number of measures including mental speed and cognitive ability.[12] Other studies have shown that meditation can improve attention, memory, and academic performance.

A number of explanations have been purposed for the cognitive benefits of meditation. So and Orme-Johnson describe meditation as a "wakeful hypometabolic" state. This state is associated with stress reduction. Meditation reduces heart rate, blood pressure, and lowers the level of the stress hormone cortisol. There is also evidence that meditation in-creases the production of brain-derived neurotrophic factor (BDNF). BDNF encourages the growth of neurons in the brain and its increase during meditation offers a plausible explanation for why some brain structures might be larger in meditators. Autopsies of people with Alzheimer's disease show that they have lower levels of BDNF in their brains.[13] This raises the interesting possibility that meditation might reduce the risk of Alzheimer's disease. Unfortunately, studies that could test this conjuncture have not yet been conducted.

Meditation has been shown to increase blood flow to the areas of the brain that regulate attention and, as we have seen, attention is a prerequisite for memory. Many meditation techniques include concentrating on a single stimulus, such as the breath or a repeated mantra. Perhaps this training in focused concentration also improves attention.

At the time of this writing I have meditated almost every day for a year and a half and I have practiced yoga every day for many years. Has yoga and meditation improved my memory? While I believe I profit from these practices, I caution the reader to take all anecdotal claims, mine or anyone else's, with a grain of salt. I could be mistaken, deluded, or lying. Once again we need to examine the research literature for clarity.

Another problem with research on meditation and yoga is that is hard to distinguish which elements of the practice actually causes the observed improvements. Yoga includes physical postures, breathing techniques, and meditation. Do all three have to be present for there to be an effect or is only one component the source of benefit? We simply don't know.

Take, for example, yogic breathing. One technique is nadhi suddhi or alternate nasal breathing. According to tradition this procedure "brings lightness of body, alertness of the mind, good appetite, proper digestion, and sound sleep." One must be properly skeptical of any such claim. After all in the same book Swami Satchidananda tells us, citing ancient authority, that through the practice of breath control "death and decay can be overcome."[14] Swami Satchidananda died in 2002.

Skeptical, but with an open mind. There have been some studies of alternate nasal breathing and the findings suggest both a potential benefit and hint at a scientific explanation. For example, Shirley Telles and her colleagues found that two yoga breathing techniques; right nasal breathing and alternative nasal breathing improved performance on a test of concentration and attention. So while the benefit may be more modest than some have claimed, it does appear to be real.

There is no shortage of good instructional material on meditation. I would suggest the writings of Vietnamese Zen Buddhist monk Thich Nhat Hanh a good place to start.

Exercise and Diet

Maintaining good physical health through exercise and diet strengthens memory and reduces your risk of dementia. A daily program of aerobic exercise and a healthy plant diet are essential components of memory improvement.[15]

[1] Dean, R. S., & Kulhavy, R. W. (1981). Influence of spatial organization in prose learning. *Journal of Educational Psychology, 73*, 57 - 64.

[2] Bellezza, F. S. (1983). The spatial arrangement of information. *Journal of Educational Psycholoy, 75*, 830 -837.

[3] Buzan, T. & Buzan, B. (1993). *The mind map book.* New York: Plume Books.

[4] Wickelgren, W. A. (1977). *Learning and memory.* Englewood Cliffs, NJ: Prentice-Hall Inc.

[5] Rasch, B. & Born, J. (2008). Reactivation and

consolidation of memory during sleep. *Current Directions in Psychological Science, 17,* 188 - 192.

[6] Vargas, J. S. (2009). *Behavior analysis for effective teaching.* New York: Routledge.

[7] Cohen, G. (1990). Why is it difficult to put names to faces? *British Journal of Psychology, 81*(3), 287-297.

[8] Feynman, R. (1974). Cargo Cult Science. *Engineering and Science, 37*(7), 10 - 13. (p. 12).

[9] Bhaskarananda, S. (2002). *The essentials of Hinduism. A comprehensive overview of the world's oldest religion.* East Seattle, WA: The Vendanta Society of Western Washington.

[10] Ospina, M. B. (2008). *Meditation practices for health: state of the research.* Rockville, MD: DIANE Publishing.

[11] Luders, E, Toga, A. W., Lepore, N., & Gaser, C. (2009). The underlying anatomical correlates of long-term meditation: Larger hippocampal and frontal volumes of gray matter. *NeuroImage, 45,* 672 – 678.

[12] So, K, & Orme-Johnson, D. W. (2001). Three randomized experiments on the longitudinal effects of the Transcendental Meditation technique on cognition. *Intelligence, 29,* 419 – 440.

[13] Phillips, H. S., Hains, J. M., Armanini, M., Laramee, G. R., Johnson, S. A., & Winslow, J. W. (1991). BDNF mRNA is decreased in the hippocampus of individuals with Alzheimer's disease. *Neuron, 7*(5), 695-702.

[14] Satchidananda, (1970). *Integral hatha yoga.* New York: Holt. (p. 144). (p. 150).

[15] Barnard, N. (2013). *Power Foods for the Brain: An Effective 3-step Plan to Protect Your Mind and Strengthen Your Memory.* New York: Hachette Digital, Inc..

Chapter 11

Memory Science and the New Mental Discipline

The Autobiography of John Stuart Mill is a fascinating account of his role as pupil in an educational experiment. James Mill, the father of John, oversaw his son's education and acted as his son's personal tutor. Central to his learning was mastery of the classical languages, Greek and Latin. Young John Stuart began studying Greek at age three and added Latin at age eight.[1]

James Mill was not alone in making Latin and Greek the center of education. The literature and language of ancient Greece and Rome were at the center of elite English education until 1918.[2]

On a practical the level the study of Latin was once important because it was the common language of European intellectuals. Great thinkers, including Issac Newton and Baruch Spinoza, wrote in Latin, not in their native tongues. Latin and Greece also became important in the Renaissance as a way to break the hold of Medieval ideas and reconnect with the values of Classical civilization. John Stuart Mill wrote in 1859 that we could "hardly be too often reminded that there was once a man called Socrates."[3]

Over time the rationale for learning these ancient languages began to change. As philosophers, theologians, and other intellectuals began writing in vernacular languages the utility of Latin as a means of communication faded. Latin, however, continued as part of the curriculum because its study was seen as a way to train the mind.

There is controversy over the origins of the modern notion of education as a kind of mind training. Some cite John Locke, some historians of education believe that the roots of formal discipline lie in the teachings of Swiss educational reformer Johann Heinrich Pestalozzi, who advocated as system of sense training. A more likely candidate is the faculty psychology that was dominate until the end of the 19th century. The faculty here refers to the many separate abilities of the mind, such as reason and memory. The mind was seen as composed of modules, and it was generally held that each module could become stronger through use.

This doctrine of formal discipline was influential in the United States during the late 19th and early 20th centuries and still has its advocates. Writing in 1905, F. C. Lewis of Dartmouth College defined formal discipline as the belief that "the study of a special subject (such as Latin) develops the powers of faculties of the mind not simply for that subject, but for any subject, however far removed and for any vocation."[4] The special subjects that were said to have these benefits included Greek, Latin and mathematics, especially Euclidean geometry.

In a survey conducted in 1903 of principals and Latin teachers in New England, Lewis found that 70% strongly endorsed the notion of formal discipline. Typical responses included "certainly the Latin students have acquired a greater power of concentration of attention, and this is of course most serviceable in the mastery of other subjects" and "Latin trains the memory."[5]

The doctrine of formal discipline is just one variety of the theory of mental discipline. There was considerable disagreement among advocates of mental discipline. Walter Kolesnik distinguishes between a conservative approach, invested in classical language and mathematics (formal discipline) and a liberal approach. The liberal version of mental discipline advocated modern subjects, especially the sciences, as a means of mental training. Thus, one must be careful here, if one version of mental discipline were disproved, it would not disprove some other form of mental training. To evaluate claims about the different forms of mental discipline we need to know something about a broader phenommenon called transfer.[6]

Transfer is a technical term used by educational psychologists to describe how learning in the past affects both performance and learning in the future. We would like to believe that learning math in the classroom would allow a student to make change when later employed as a cashier. We expect that the skills taught in English class will help a student complete a job application or write a report at work. We also expect old learning to help new learning. Sometimes, this preparatory value of past learning is obvious. Learning algebra skills certainly helps us master calculus. In any kind of sequential material, where learning step B depends upon learning step A, we could say a kind of transfer of learning is involved. Clearly learning to read in the elementary grades helps us learn material from textbooks later on.

There are also times when past learning interferes with new learning, a phenomenon called negative transfer. Those who learned how to drive with a manual transmission note the difficulties they have when they try to learn how to drive an automatic. Frequently they try to step on a clutch that isn't there and "ghost shift" at inappropriate times.

Another way to think about the effects of negative transfer is to imagine trying to learn a new system of touch typing. The standard arrangement of keys on your computer is called QWERTY, it is named after the 6 letters keys running above your left hand. There is debate about the history and efficiency of this arrangement of keys, for our purposes all you need to know is that alternative key arrangements exist. Let us assume, as their inventors and partisans insist, that these alternative systems of typing allow for faster typing. Would you switch? Just thinking about the difficulty of making such a change is headache inducing. Here negative transfer has produced a path dependency; the death of the old system would require nothing less than the passing of an entire generation and its replacement with young people trained exclusively in the new way.

So the effects of transfer can be powerful. Indeed, our usual expectation is that skills learned in school will transfer into to a broad range of contexts.

Implicit in the idea of mental discipline is a notion about how we might harness the power of transfer. Mental discipline argues that it might be possible to train our mental capacities to operate more efficiently across some broad range of tasks.[7] Formal discipline goes one step further and identifies specific subject areas, Latin, Greek, and, sometimes, mathematics, as having special powers to train the mind. Thus, the advocates of formal discipline reason that these subjects should be at the core of the curriculum.

Mental discipline and formal discipline have been controversial for over one hundred years, and the debate continues today.

Indeed, the claim of general transfer has been taken up by many teachers seeking to preserve their discipline in the face of school funding cuts. We often hear that music or art will improve your scores on standardized tests. Some of the claims seem more plausible than others. Kolesnik documents a claim made in 1867 that heraldry, the study of family coats of arms, had benefits as a form of mental discipline.[8] The most extravagant recent claim I have heard in this regard was from a fencing coach who claimed that fencing could improve math performance. Apparently she is not alone. An article by reporter Ernest Scheyder, of the Columbia News Service tells us to "take up fencing" if we find math difficult.[9] Fencing, we are told, involves geometry and timing, and we should be able to transfer these skills to the math classroom. While there is a certain charm in this and one wishes it to be true, the author and his sources present no evidence.

I do not know of any research evidence that confirms the mental training effects of fencing or even, for that matter, heraldry. One should always have an open mind and be willing to wait for evidence. On the other hand, it seems unfortunate that teachers feel that they have to make such justifications. There are many things that enrich our lives and should be taught even if they cannot be captured on an achievement test. Art, music, and literature have value in of and of themselves. They may not make us more employable, but they make us better people.

What about the study of Latin?

Latin learning has been shown to have some specific transfer effects. It will certainly help you in areas of study such as law and anatomy that rely on Latinate vocabulary and it seems to help students master the academic vocabulary. Thus, learning Latin does have some specific transfer effects.[10] General transfer seems more elusive. There is little evidence that Latin helps us think more logically. We should not, however, allow ourselves to misled by inferring relative worth from the distinction between specific transfer and general transfer. While Latin's effect on general vocabulary skills may be characterized as specific transfer, its benefits are still large.

However, it should be noted that vocabulary benefits can be derived from direct study of vocabulary. There are a number of vocabulary programs that focus on learning word roots and affixes that have been shown to improve vocabulary.

Thus, we see that there is more than a grain of truth in some of the claims of formal discipline; there is a general vocabulary capacity that we can train directly, and this capacity has great benefits in school and in life. Are there other kinds of mental discipline besides formal discipline that might have great transfer powers? My assertion here is that memory training can become the new mental discipline. This is a controversial claim. Many have argued that it is not possible to train the memory. Let us look at the evidence.

One of the earliest experiments in memory training was conducted by William James using himself as a subject. In eight daily sessions, he memorized the first 158 lines of Victor Hugo's poem *Satyr*. It took him 131.83 minutes to memorize the poem. Unlike Ebbinghaus he does not give us a clear definition of his criterion for memorization. Then, working for 20 minutes a day, he memorized the entire first book of *Paradise Lost*. This took him 38 days.

In order to see if all this daily practice with memorization improved his memory, he learned the next 158 lines of *Satyr*. Once again he worked over 8 daily sessions but this time it took him 151.5 minutes to learn the poem. From his calculation, he had gone from a learning rate of one line per 50 seconds to one line per 57 seconds. His memory practice had not helped him.

Not satisfied with his results, James persuaded several people to repeat his experiments. The results were mixed; some found improvements others had outcomes similar to those found by James. There were variations in the experimental procedures so it is difficult to draw a general conclusion from these experiments.

One of James' collaborator, William H. Burnham, suggested that the study be conducted using nonsense syllables, like those used by Ebbinghaus. James persuaded two students to do this. Unfortunately, the records of the experiment were lost and James can only tell us "the result was a very considerable shortening of the average time of the second series of nonsense-syllables, learned after training."[11] From the description provided by James, which is not very clear, it seems that the students tested themselves on nonsense syllables, but trained themselves memorizing poetry. If so, this would be an impressive result. The use of nonsense syllables would have partially controlled for the difficulty and associability of both the pre-training and post-training material. This control was not in place for his other experiments. James speculates that the improvement may have been caused by a process of habituation to nonsense syllables. This would seem unlikely since the students only used nonsense words on the pre and post tests. Thus, on the most rigorous test he describes memory training did seem to improve memory.

James gives us one more anecdote, the case of a minister who recorded how long it took him to memorize a sermon over the course of his career. Before the age of 20, it took him four days to memorize a one hour sermon. Over time the interval needed for memorization fell to 2 days, then half a day, and, finally, to one hour.[12]

Since James did not take the same care as Ebbinghaus or later researchers it is hard to interpret his results. For example, we do not even know if the first 158 lines of the poem he used in his pre-test were as difficult as the subsequent 158 lines he used in his post-test. Moreover, the procedures used in the several replications he described were not consistent. Thus, the results are hard to compare. Given the poor quality of these data it is surprising that they are often cited as proof that you cannot improve memory through practice. A greater surprise is that less than a decade after James reported that he could not improve his memory for poetry by practice he wrote, "learning poetry by heart will make it easier to learn and remember poetry, but nothing else."[13]

What is even more surprising is that when you read the many efforts to replicate these results, the research is inconsistent. Some studies find that memory training produces substantial memory improvement, and others could find no benefit.[14]

Some have claimed that it is possible to train memory for a particular area, but not to improve memory as a general faculty. If you practice memorizing poetry, your ability to memorize poetry might increase. For example, a study conducted by Kate Gordon in 1933 found that student's ability to memorize Shakespeare's sonnets improved with practice.[15] While the ability to memorize poetry may itself be a worthy goal, this argument claims there is no evidence that it will improve your memory in general. Memory of poetry increases your knowledge base about the nature of poetry and, thus, may make it easier to learn new poetry. This is not because your memory as a general faculty has improved. Your memory is not like a muscle that improves with exercise, rather it improves with expertise.[16] Thus, expert chess players improve their memory for chess, but that does not generalize to general overall improvement.

However, there are studies that show that memory training does, at least sometimes, generalize to other areas. One of the most interesting studies in this regard, was conducted by Herbert Woodrow of the University of Minnesota. Woodrow used a variety of memory tests, including memory for poetry, prose, facts, dates and vocabulary. He divided the participants, all university sophomores, into 3 groups: a control group that only took the pretest and the post-test and two memory groups.

These two groups were both told that they would be receiving memory training. However, the nature of the training was very different. While both groups practiced using nonsense syllables, one group was taught to practice rote memorization. The other group was a taught a variety of memory strategies and then practiced using these strategies to memorize material. These memory techniques included self-testing, and forming associations. Both groups had eight training sessions, and the time for each session was the same.

Contrary to James' experiment, the group that only practiced rote memory of poetry did show some improvement. However, the improvement was small. On the other hand, the group that was taught memory techniques and given the opportunity to practice them showed substantial improvement in memory abilities on the final test.[17]

Why might it be the case that memory is improved in some training experiments and not in others? I think the difference may lie in what is being trained. If we cast our mind back to the experiment conducted by Ericsson where a college student practiced memorizing strings of digits for one hour a day several days a week. After 230 hours of practice the student's ability to remember a string of random digits rose from seven to 79 digits. What was important was not the repeated practice of digit memorization, but the repeated practice of memory techniques. Ericsson's work suggests that memory could be improved through the practice of memory strategies. [18] Thus, the study and application of memory techniques is a kind of mental discipline.

Based on his poetry experiment and his reading of the literature William James came to the conclusion that:

> there can be no improvement of the general or elementary faculty of memory; there can only be improvement of our memory for special systems of associated things; and the latter improvement is due to the way in which the things in question are woven into association with each other in the mind. Intricately woven or profoundly woven, they are held; disconnected, they tend to drop out just in proportion as the native brain retentiveness is poor.[19]

What James misses here is that while rote memorization practice may have little value, there are techniques, such as the mnemonic strategies that can improve with practice. Unfortunately, because of his prestige, James rejection of memory practice stifled this area in both research and practice.

The general principles and techniques we have discussed in this book constitute a special set of skills that, once learned, can be applied in many learning contexts. Memory techniques, including the use of mnemonics, the spacing effect and the testing effect, can be applied across the curriculum and in life outside of school. In 1988, psychologist Frank Dempster, bemoaned the fact that the spacing effect, a phenomenon well established by research, had not been applied to classroom learning.[20] Over a quarter of a century later, there is little evidence that this situation has changed. Indeed, I suspect most teachers today have never even heard of the spacing effect or many of the other memory improvement techniques I have described in this book.

One obvious example, an approach that could be easily applied in classrooms, is the 3R (Read, Recite, and Read) technique, described in Chapter 9. Psychologists have demonstrated the effectiveness of 3R. They noted that 3R is "portable to all learning settings, both formal and informal."[21] Teachers should be taught and be expected to teach 3R.

A thorough grounding in memory for students and teachers would have enormous positive benefits. It would allow students to improve their achievement in all subjects. It would also help them increase their fluency in basic skills and provide a secure footing for higher order pursuits. These techniques reduce the burden of memorization, they allow students to learn more material in a shorter period of time.

Language learning researcher Jan Hulstijn advocates direct instruction of mnemonics in language classrooms telling us "time spent on confrontation with the vocabulary learning problem in such a metacogntitive way is time well spent."[22] He goes on to point out that we need to remind students repeatedly to use mnemonics so that they acquire the habit of using these techniques. I think this is good advice for all classes, the scaffolding and direct instruction of memory techniques should be an expected part of teaching.

Memory Improvement is Liberating

Memory work can be drudgery, but it also can be joyous. To memorize a favorite poem, or a speech from a play, is to have intimate knowledge of it. To know some fact about the world with precision allows us to reason and think creatively.

Philosopher and essayist Jim Holt has written on the deep pleasures that come from memorizing poetry. According to Holt, after he has memorized a poem he becomes "the possessor of a nice big piece of poetical real estate, one that I will always be able to revisit and roam about in."[23]

Memory is a wonderful faculty. It remains at the core of what it means to be an educated person. Memory improvement is desirable and possible. It should be a core part of education. Let us embrace this new mental discipline.

---

[1] Mill, J. S. (1957/1873). *Autobiography*. Indianapolis, IN: Bobbs-Merrill Educational Publishing.

[2] Oglivie, R. M. (1964). *Latin and Greek: A history of the influence of the classics on English life from 1600 to 1918*. London: Routledge and Kegan Paul

[3] Mill, J. S.(1859). *On liberty*. London: John W. Parker and Son. (p. 46).

[4] Lewis, F. C. (1905). A study in formal discipline. *The School Review, 13*, 281 - 292. (p. 282).

[5] Lewis, F. C. (1905). A study in formal discipline. *The School Review, 13*, 281 - 292. (p. 281).

[6] Kolesnik, W. B. (1958). *Mental discipline and modern education.* Madison, WI: University of Wisconsin Press.

[7] Kolesnik, W. B. (1958). *Mental discipline and modern education.* Madison, WI: University of Wisconsin Press.

[8] Kolesnik, W. B. (1958). *Mental discipline and modern education.* Madison, WI: University of Wisconsin Press.

[9] Scheyder, E. (2007, April 14). Have problems with math? Take up fencing! *The Indianan Gazette,* (p. E2).

[10] Masciantonio, R. (1977). Tangible benefits of the study of Latin: A review of research. *Foreign Language Annals, 10*(4), 375-382.

[11] James, W. (1890/1950). *The Principles of Psychology.* New York: Dover Publications. (p. 667).

[12] James, W. (1890/1950). *The Principles of Psychology.* New York: Dover Publications

[13] James, W. (1899/1958). *Talks to teachers: On psychology; and to students on some of life's ideals.* New York: W. W. Norton & Company. (p. 94).

[14] Kolesnik, W. B. (1958). *Mental discipline and modern education.* Madison, WI: University of

Wisconsin Press.

[15] Gordon, K. (1933). Some records of the memorizing of sonnets. *Journal of Experimental Psychology,16,* 701-708.

[16] Radvansky, G. A. (2011). *Human memory.* Boston; Allyn & Bacon.

[17] Woodrow, H. (1927). The effect of training upon transference. *Journal of Educational Psychology, 18,* 159 - 172.

[18] Ericsson, K. A., & Chase, W. G., (1982). Exceptional memory. *American Scientist, 70,* 607 – 615.

[19] James, W. (1899/1958). *Talks to teachers: On psychology; and to students on some of life's ideals.* New York: W. W. Norton & Company. (pp. 90 - 91).

[20] Dempster, F. N. (1988). The spacing effect: A case study in the failure to apply the results of psychological research. *American Psychologist, 43,* 627 - 634.

[21] McDaniel, , M. A., Howard, D. C., and Einstein, G. O., (2009). The read-recite-review study strategy: Effective and portable. *Psychological Science, 20,* 516 - 522. (p. 516).

[22] Hulstijn, J. H. (1997). Mnemonic methods in foreign language vocabulary learning: Theoretical considerations and pedagogical implications. In J. Coady & T. Huckin (Eds.). *Second language vocabulary acquisition: A rationale for pedagogy.*

(pp. 203 - 224). Cambridge, UK: Cambridge University Press. (p. 217).

[23] Holt, J. (April 5, 2009). Got poetry? *The New York Times.* (p. BR23)

Appendix
My Memory Workout

Here is my daily memory workout.

1. Five to ten minutes of study spaced repetition software. I use Anki (available at http://ankisrs.net/). Anki allows me to enter in any material I want to incorporate into my long term memory. For example, every time I see a movie or read a book I enter the title into Anki. For example, I might enter the prompt "film about British pensioners living in an Indian Hotel," with the answer "The Best Exotic Marigold Hotel." This makes it more likely that I will be able to recall the titles of films and books in conversation.

I enter into Anki any piece of information that I find interesting or feel that I might like to recall at a later date. When reading books, I note interesting facts that I wish to retrain and write the page number on the inside front cover or on a bookmark. When I'm finished with the book, I'll enter those facts into Anki.

When possible I add photographs of people whose names I might like to recall as a prompt. I also put in the photos of movie stars, celebrities, politicians, and people from history whose names I don't want to forget.

Finally, I add to Anki any material that I have had a recent tip of the tongue experience. So I have added a photo of Willie Nelson as a prompt to help me remember his name.

2. Five minutes of work with Memrise (available at http://www.memrise.com/). I use Memrise to learn foreign language vocabularies.

3. One half hour of treadmill language study. I walk on a treadmill for one hour every morning during one half hour of that time I study languages. I either listen to interactive language programs such as Pimsleur or review flash cards.

Walking is an excellent way to stay fit, which, in turn will reduce your risk of dementia and many other health problems.

4. Meditation. I practice at least fifteen minutes of meditation every day. There are many kinds of meditation, I have found metta meditation works best for me, but I suggest you experiment with a number of approaches when you begin, settling on one over time.

I found that guided meditation recordings were helpful at first; they helped me get used to the daily discipline of sitting, but, eventually, I came to find them distracting and stopped using them.

One piece of meditation technology that I adopted and continue to use is the Insight Timer, available as a smartphone app. Insight Timer tracks your daily meditation and acts as a social network with other meditators. It is an excellent motivator.

5. Yoga. I make time to practice yoga every day. If I am able, I go to a studio for an intensive class but if not I always practice a few poses every day.

6. I eat a well balanced plant based diet with lots of green leafy vegetables, fruits, and whole grains. I rely on the nonprofit website NutrionFacts.org website,

run by Dr. Michael Greger, for research based nutrition information.